Singing Groups for people with Dementia

Singing Groups for people with Dementia

A guide to setting up and running groups in community and residential settings

DIANA KERR

THE CHOIR PRESS

First published in the United Kingdom in 2015 by
The Choir Press

ISBN 978-1-909300-95-8

Without understanding music theory,
we can appreciate music as pleasure or art.
Without knowing, we Dance.
Without understanding, we Sing.
Without learning, we Know.

John M Ortiz from the *The Tao of Music.*

Contents

Acknowledgements

So many people have contributed to this book it seems wrong to pick out a few. There are, however, people who must be acknowledged.

Sheila Hardie, without whom the book would never have come into being. It was she who persuaded me to 'put my money where my mouth was' and get involved in setting up a singing group for people with dementia. Sheila and the other two members of the triumvirate, Kate Walker and Pam Robertson, have been invaluable companions along the road.

Annabelle Meredith, who, many years ago, showed me the power of music with people with dementia, has been and continues to be a source of inspiration.

Meg Adams, who has encouraged and cajoled when I needed it and made really helpful suggestions.

May Ross and Brian Kerr, who have both edited and encouraged and listened to endless chat from me about the book.

Bob Simans, Nilanjana Maulik, Geraldine Lloyd, Brian Hardie, Alan Midwinter and all the other people, volunteers, staff, families, friends and members of singing groups who have both entertained and informed me.

Introduction

When I tell people about using music with people with dementia, and in particular when I tell them about my own involvement in a singing group for people with dementia and their carers, I am usually met with great enthusiasm. I then hear, 'But how do you go about doing it?', 'What do I need to know to set up a group?', 'I am not really very musical but I would like to do it,' or even, 'I'm tone deaf, so I could not do it.'

The purpose of this book is to try to answer the above questions and to demystify any ideas there may be about using music for and with people with dementia. It is to encourage everyone who thinks that they would like to have a go at using music in this way.

Of course before having a go there are things that need to be known and put in place. My own experience is that there is quite a lot to know and a need for good preparation and long-term planning. Starting a group either in the community or in a residential home, nursing home or day centre requires more than some songs and enthusiasm, although, of course, both these things are essential. If the preparation and forward planning are not in place there is a danger that the enterprise will be short-lived and everyone will be disappointed. Hopefully this book will help to equip you with the knowledge that you need to make a success of your undertaking.

The focus of the book is on setting up and running singing groups where the emphasis is on people having a good old sing-song. It is not about setting up a choir. There are choirs for people with dementia, but these require a different focus, commitment, skill and involvement from people with dementia. Choirs, of necessity, will have more emphasis on getting things right. There is also a potential conflict of interest when the progression of the dementia means that people are not able to fulfil the requirements and are faced with another loss.

This is also definitely not about organising singers and choirs to come into homes and perform. The purpose of the groups described in this book is for people to be active participants and not passive receivers of entertainment. Whilst there is clearly a place for being entertained, the activities described in this book have a different purpose and outcome.

The book is divided into three parts.

Part One, 'Music and Dementia: What You Need to Know', has chapters on why music is so important to everyone and why it is particularly important to people with dementia. There is a chapter on dementia which provides important information about dementia and how it affects people.

Part Two, 'Preparing to Get Started', has chapters on how to prepare yourself and others. This part will address issues such as what people need to know and do, what to look for in a venue, how to advertise the group, what equipment might be needed and, where appropriate, what needs to be considered in setting up a committee and having a constitution.

Part Three, 'Planning, Organising and Running Sessions', deals with the session content and structure. Information about where and how to access songs and music is given. Reasons for using different songs and different song formats are given along with sample programmes.

There are many books and articles on the subject of using music with people with dementia (Aldridge, 2000; Clair, 1996; Clair, 1991), but most are written by music therapists and academics and are essentially for other music therapists and academics. The intention in this book is to go a bit further and show that you do not need to be a music therapist or indeed an accomplished musician to use music. This does not mean that musical knowledge is not a great help, and for some of the activities we describe there will be a need for a certain level of musical know-how and skill, but that is not necessarily what is needed. If that becomes an essential criterion then many opportunities to use music will be missed.

The focus in this book is on using music in groups rather than in an individual therapy session where the intention is more about reaching an individual with specific needs.

If you are thinking about using music with people with dementia then hopefully this book will encourage, inform and enthuse you. Good luck.

PART ONE

Music and Dementia: What You Need to Know

CHAPTER ONE

What is so good about music?

Desert Island Discs

Desert Island Discs is a programme on BBC Radio 4 that has been running since 1942. The format of the programme is that the interviewee recounts, chronologically, events in their lives and selects eight records that either reflect on the events or have some significant meaning to them in relation to an event, memory or person. The power of the music to evoke the past for them and to convey to the listener the meaning and emotion for the interviewee is no doubt one of the reasons why this is such a popular programme. Its longevity is testimony to the fact that it touches such important aspects of people's lives. It is a wonderful example of the power of music to evoke memory, communicate emotion and make links across the airwaves to unknown listeners. The music selected is for and about the interviewee, but it resonates with the millions of listeners who will often attach their own emotions and memories to the music.

Everyone responds to music; even the people I referred to in the introduction who say they are tone deaf. They are not tone deaf but have just not trained themselves to listen to, and adjust, their voices. Often they are people who were told at school not to join the choir because they were not singing in tune at the time.

'Music, in its many and various forms, exists and is central in every culture' (Sacks, 2007). It varies from one culture to another but, in a way, that shows how central it is. It reflects something about each culture and you can often hear the culture in the music. Think of Spanish flamenco music, Chinese songs and Welsh choirs, Hindi songs and English folk songs: how different and reflective of their culture and time they are. No matter what the culture, the music is reflecting and moving its audience.

Humans are a musical species as Oliver Sacks (2007) says: 'All of us (with very few exceptions) can perceive music, perceive tones, timbre, pitch intervals, melodic contours, harmony and (perhaps most elementally) rhythm.' You may not know the meaning of all the terms he uses but that does not mean you cannot make and appreciate the music, and that is what is important.

The fact that music is somehow an integral part of being human is perhaps best illustrated by the response of babies and their mothers to music. New mothers, unprompted, will hum and sing to their infant knowing that that is likely to soothe and calm them. The baby's response to music may be partly because they have already heard this in the womb; the sound of the mother's heartbeat (a basic and well-used rhythm) will already be familiar as a foundation for music appreciation and response. Very early on, babies start to spontaneously vocalise; the sounds that they make really do seem like early attempts to sing, and soon they will begin to incorporate sounds around them and to extend their range. By the time they are two, children will show a preference for the music of their own culture.

During our teens we begin to identify personal musical preferences, and as adults the music that we seem to be nostalgic for and to remember best is the music of our teenage years. This is probably partly because adolescence is a time of heightened emotion and we tend to remember things that have heightened emotional content. Since music during our teens is often expressing emotions that are hard to articulate, it is not surprising that these are the memories that stick. Also, as Levitin (2006) writes, 'it is around fourteen that the wiring of our musical brains is approaching adultlike levels of completion.' Whatever the reason, the music of those years is the music we remember well.

Our response to music can, of course, run the whole gamut of our emotions. We will often choose music to reflect our mood. If we are feeling down we will listen to music that reinforces the mood and in a way gives us even more strength to wallow and sigh; think of the lovesick youth. Conversely we will use music to lift our spirits and express our joy.

It is almost as if we are hard-wired to use and respond to music. The power of music to evoke emotions and influence our feelings about things is understood well by advertisers who will employ music to heighten our response to, and so our liking or even craving for, inanimate objects such as cars, clothes, food and drink and even the latest electronic device.

An important element of music is that it has a pulse; remember the mother's heartbeat that is the first pulse the baby hears. Levitin (2007) says that most music is foot-tapping. He states 'we listen to music that has a pulse, something you can tap your foot to, or at least tap the foot in your mind to'. I am not sure if much foot tapping goes on when listening to a Beethoven sonata or a Bach cantata, but the point he is making is that listening to music involves our bodies and something physical happens. Nietzsche (1888) maintained that we listen to music with our muscles. He was right. We resonate to the music; it gets into our bodies as well as our minds. Our bodies respond to music. We keep time, perhaps by simply tapping our feet, or maybe by moving to the beat when we dance or march. We can even respond unwittingly. People doing workouts in the gym can change their rate of running, jumping or whatever activity it is they are doing if the music they are listening to is changed. The person exercising may not be conscious of the change, but their body is.

So music gets to us emotionally and physically, even to those people who maintain that they are tone deaf. The very few people who do not respond to music are likely to be suffering from a rare condition. Music gets underneath our skin and as Schopenhauer (1819/1996) asserted, 'The inexplicable depth of music ... is due to the fact that it reproduces all the emotions of our innermost being'.

A good way to illustrate what is so good about music and the way in which it is in all of our lives is for you, the reader, to do the following exercise. Many of you may have done this already.

Pretend you are on *Desert Island Discs* and think of eight discs you would want to have with you if you were stranded on a desert island. List each piece of music and think about why you chose it, what memories it holds and what emotions it evokes. Which one would you keep if you could only have one of the eight?

Listening to music is undeniably an emotional and physical experience which enhances and enriches our lives. Creating our own music, either through singing or through playing, adds another layer to the enjoyment and personal involvement. Playing and singing with other people, however, adds a whole new dimension to the emotional and physical experience.

The level of enjoyment can be quite exhilarating. Singing releases feel-good hormones, endorphins and the anxiety-busting hormone oxytocin. It is a stress reducer, so it is not surprising that research has found that singing together not only improves your sense of wellbeing but is actually good for your health. Beck et al. (2000) found that being a member of a choir improved the immune systems of the singers. There is evidence that singing in a choir affects our heart rate; choirs have been shown to synchronise their heart and breathing rates, increasing and decreasing them in response to the music (Vickhoff et al., 2013). Singing together also appears to help reduce high blood pressure (Valentine and Evans, 2001).

In addition, during singing and making music a series of connections are made in the brain, and if these are accessed regularly this helps our creativity and our problem-solving skills (Noice et al., 2013; Welch et al., 2010).

Singing on your own is good for you and, so long as you do not have anxieties about performance, singing in groups is even better.

CHAPTER TWO

What is so good about music for people with dementia?

The previous chapter made clear why and how music is profoundly important and a core element in all our lives.

This is no less the case for people with dementia. As other experiences become confusing and communication becomes difficult, the role and experience of music become even more important. Music stays with us long after speech and other skills have gone. Anyone who has worked with people with dementia will have witnessed the remarkable fact that people who have lost the ability to speak coherently or even at all will sing an entire song perfectly. It is not only the words but the musical memory that stays, so people will hum or whistle a tune even when the words to the song have gone.

One of the important aspects of supporting people with dementia is minimising the impact of their losses and playing to their strengths. If people can sing then we should be encouraging this, helping them maintain the skill and the sense of achievement and joy that goes with that. Even at the end stage of the condition, when people are close to death, music will reach them. It is important not to assume that the person lying inert and apparently not responding is oblivious to the sound of music. Play or sing to people at this end stage and you will see changes in their facial expression and even vocal activity and physical movement. Music can provide one last way to reach the person and enable them to respond at an emotional level.

There is a substantial body of research evidencing the crucial role that music plays in our support of people with dementia.

We know that music is effective in reducing a range of challenging behaviour. Playing calming music will reduce agitation (Denny, 1997). Music can also reduce aggressive behaviour, 'wandering', repetitive vocalisation and irritability (Groene, 1993; Casby & Holm, 1994; Ragneskog et al., 1996). This is perhaps not surprising if we recognise the calming effect that music can have.

It is important, however, to note that music should not be played for more than 20 minutes at a time as the research shows that it can become a source of irritation and cause distress. This may not always be the case, but carers need to monitor this and not just leave music playing.

We know that if caregivers sing to people with dementia when carrying out intimate tasks, the incidence of challenging behaviour can be significantly reduced. This may be the result of a number of factors. For the carer the mere act of singing reduces stress in them and this will be transmitted to the person with dementia. Also the sound of the carer singing may be calming because it is reminiscent of the mother singing to the child.

If we play the right music at mealtimes people will be more relaxed, will sit longer at the meal and will eat more (Ragneskog et al., 1996). Given that people with dementia have problems with eating, this seems to be an opportunity not to be missed. Remember to be sure that you use music that is important to the person with dementia. Different people will respond to different music. There is evidence that the music we remember best is the music that we heard between the ages of 16 and 24.

Using music appropriately can lead to an improvement in reality orientation, memory recall and social behaviour. Music will often trigger communication. It may trigger speech but it can also allow the person with dementia to sing something that reflects their mood or articulates something they want to say. I was in a residential home when a lady I know came up to me and sang 'Show Me the Way to Go Home'. She was communicating very well through her singing!

Music can awaken our connection to the world and our history, and this is true for people with dementia.

The following two stories are wonderful illustrations of this and many of the other points above.

Malcolm and Isobel

Malcolm heard of a singing group being set up in his local community for people with dementia and their carers. His wife Isobel, who had dementia, had not spoken for the last five months. She no longer showed any facial expression and seemed to be in a world of her own.

With great trepidation Malcolm brought Isobel to the group.

To begin with Isobel appeared agitated and just sat and stared as the singing got underway. Slowly her hand started to tap her thigh, then she moved her body, then she began to make some humming noises. By the end of the session Isobel was singing and smiling.

The next morning she woke up and said to her husband, 'I think we should bake a cake today,' and they did!

Kate

Kate sang in a band as a young woman and continued to sing throughout her life. Her dementia was at such a stage that conversation was limited and she did not sing at all, even with the encouragement of her family.

Her husband and daughter brought Kate to our singing group in the hope that she might sing. The singing leader that day had brought hats which resembled the hats worn by the Andrews Sisters, who were popular during the era when Kate was singing in the band. She offered the hats to anyone who might want to wear them whilst we sang 'Don't Sit Under the Apple Tree'.

With encouragement, Kate took a hat and, along with another member of the group and the singing leader, started to sing and slowly parade around the hall whilst everyone sang. It seemed that the setup had triggered memories for Kate and it became obvious that she had moved into 'performance mode'. Not only did she sing but she took a bow at the end of her 'performance'.

Needless to say, her husband and daughter shed more than a few tears.

It would be foolish and wrong to pretend that music always leads to such dramatic events. The above stories are, however, two of many that could be told, some not as dramatic but for the person involved still a very worthwhile and life-enhancing experience.

We know that singing and listening to music can make us happy. Even if the person with dementia forgets that they were singing soon after the event, this does not negate its worth. They will still feel good even if they cannot remember why. People with dementia live much in the moment, so we should be trying to make as many of their moments as possible good ones, and music undoubtedly achieves this.

If you are not using music as something to listen to, dance to, or sing along to, then people with dementia are being deprived of a wonderful, core human activity that will enrich their lives.

The following quote from a manager of a residential care home is a clear affirmation of the reasons to set up a singing group in every home:

'I am in absolutely no doubt whatsoever of the benefits derived by those residents who participate [in the music] – at least 70%! The music clearly stimulates residents and has improved, even for a short period, individual levels of self-esteem and quality of life. Residents become lively and animated, their eyes are more alert and bright and they become more expressive. Those with severe dementia appear to gain most. I am aware that the aural sense is the last sense to diminish, so it is vitally important that we keep stimulating this sense for as long as possible.'

CHAPTER THREE

What do you need to know about dementia?

Janet

> Janet was a volunteer working in a singing group in a residential home. She had volunteered after her mother had died. Her mother had had dementia. Janet had been very concerned that her mother had not had sufficient stimulation in the home she was in. She also knew that her mother loved to sing. Janet was motivated to try to make sure others had what her mother would have loved.
>
> During an early session Sally, a resident, told Janet that she was going home at the end of the session as her mother would be wondering where she was.
>
> Janet explained to Sally that this was her home now and that her mother had died some years ago.
>
> Sally became very agitated, accused Janet of lying and became very angry when she was not allowed to go home.
>
> Janet had had no training on how to respond to people with dementia and was doing what she thought was the right thing.

It is essential that everyone involved in the sessions has an understanding of the needs of people with dementia. If they do not then there is a good chance that they may say or do something that might distress, agitate or confuse a participant. As one of the main aims of the sessions is to relax people and for them to enjoy themselves, staff, volunteers and carers must get the right response and communicate in the right way.

Ideally everyone involved would receive suitable training in dementia care, but as this may not always be provided I am including information about dementia which everyone needs to read and apply.

What is dementia?

There are many different dementias, so when we say someone has dementia we are not being very precise. Dementia is a general or umbrella term used to describe a number of conditions that are damaging to the brain. The symptoms will vary slightly depending on the type of dementia and the person. No two people will have the condition in the same way. Generally, however, the person will experience a progressive deterioration in all areas of functioning.

A few of the most common types of dementia are listed here.

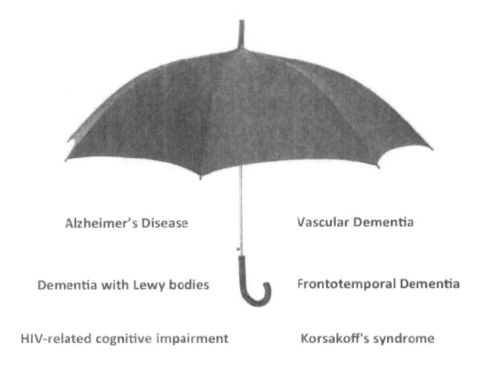

Alzheimer's Disease   Vascular Dementia

Dementia with Lewy bodies   Frontotemporal Dementia

HIV-related cognitive impairment   Korsakoff's syndrome

Creutzfeldt-Jakob disease

The most common dementia is Alzheimer's disease, followed by vascular dementia and dementia with Lewy bodies.

Additionally, although the damage is irreversible, it is characteristic of people with dementia to be more receptive some days than others and even to change throughout the course of the day. This may in part be because they are affected by things like tiredness, stress, light levels, anxiety and physical illness.

Although all dementias and people are different, there are a number of common characteristics that you may observe:

- **Failing memory.** People start to lose their short-term memory. They will forget something they did yesterday but still remember something they did years ago.
- **Loss of memory for words.** People will struggle with finding the right word and will often use another similar word instead. For example they may say 'foot thing' for 'shoe' or just 'that thing' when they cannot remember a word.
- **Impaired ability to learn new things.** People will find it increasingly hard to learn new tasks, hobbies etc.
- **High susceptibility to stress, anxiety, fear and panic.** People will become very quickly upset and anxious, often about things that to other people seem minor and not stressful. Loud noises, being contradicted and being asked questions will be very stressful.
- **Changes in mood, personality and behaviour.** Traits may become exaggerated or diminished. A gregarious person may become more so or may become surprisingly quiet.
- **Impaired reasoning.** Decreasing ability to reason things out means that people will often make wrong assumptions. If they cannot find something then, rather than use reason to work though where or how they might have misplaced it, they will accuse someone of stealing it.
- **Difficulty with purposeful movements.** People will have problems with doing things in a set order and particularly with organising physical activities which involve the purposeful use of their bodies. Touching specific parts of their body, clapping, sitting down and so on can become a problem.

- **Acute sensitivity to the social and built environment.** People will find many environments too noisy and too busy. They may think shiny floors in toilets are water and they will have difficulty remembering where rooms such as toilets are. They will also see changes in colour on the floor as changes in height. You will see people trying to step over things that are not there just because of changes in floor colour.

Having read all the above you will see that people with dementia are struggling to cope; they feel lost, can easily become anxious and often feel threatened by the unknown. A core tenet of being with and supporting people with dementia is:

DO NOT STRESS THEM.

This is easier said than done but, if you are trying to decide what to say or do with someone with dementia, always try to choose the thing that will not stress them.

One of the things you will have noticed about people with dementia is that they cannot remember recent things and yet can remember things from the distant past. Very often they appear to have a different reality to the rest of us.

This can be the cause of much distress for everyone involved.

Peter

> Peter, a man of 88, had a diagnosis of dementia. He had been married to his second wife for 38 years. He, however, insisted that she was a stranger to him and, although he tolerated her in the house in the day when he saw her as a cleaner, he was aggressive and distressed at night when she would not leave and go home.
>
> Understandably this was very distressing for his wife.

To understand the difficulties that people with dementia experience in relation to their memory and understanding of where they are, what they are doing and who they and others are, it is necessary to understand some of the ways in which memory is stored and subsequently damaged by the dementia.

When someone develops dementia, they have increasing difficulty learning new things and even lose the ability to retain the memory they have. As the dementia progresses, even information and events that are stored in the long-term memory will begin to disappear.

Huub Buijssen (2005) describes and illustrates this process through the idea of diaries. He describes our memory as stored in diaries, one for each year of our life. People without dementia will have all their diaries stored chronologically and intact on the shelf.

If we imagine a shelf of diaries, one diary for each year of our life, then with the onset of dementia memories begin to get lost and a domino effect takes place with the diaries slowly falling down. Only those left standing will have meaning and memory for us. Buijssen describes this as roll-back memory.

Below is an excellent illustration of this process, taken directly from Buijssen (2005):

The memory of a 77-year-old without dementia – the shelf on which the diaries containing the memories of his entire life are stacked is still intact.

Years

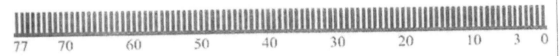

The memory of a 77-year-old patient with dementia who has lost his memories of the last 17 years – the diaries begin to collapse, first the most recent, then those preceding them, and so on.

Years

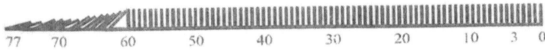

The memory of someone in the advanced stage of dementia – only the memories of his early childhood remain.

Years

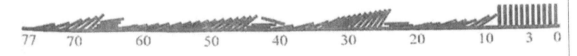

Buijssen, H (2005), The Simplicity of Dementia, London: Jessica Kingsley Publishers, p. 37. Copyright © Huub Buijssen

This shows how people with dementia will experience themselves as younger and will forget events and people in the more recent past. This means that people begin to lose the ability to recognise the familiar. They may well perceive the world as a foreign place peopled by strangers, and the consequence is that their reality becomes different to ours. It is important to remember that their reality is as real to them as ours is to us.

This roll-back memory also helps to explain why people with dementia are so fond of songs from their past. These will be in their diaries that are still intact.

If we fail to appreciate the way in which our response to a person with dementia can exacerbate the feelings of fear, confusion, anger and loss then we will only make things worse.

There are lots of things you need to know about helping people with dementia, but the remit of this book means that only a limited amount can be covered. I would, however, recommend that everyone watch the excellent video *Darkness in the Afternoon*, which can be obtained from the Dementia Services Development Centre at the University of Stirling.

Below I have listed a number of things that you need to be aware of when communicating and being with people with dementia.

Things you need to do:

- Be patient.
- Sit at eye level when talking to the person.
- Hold their hand if appropriate when communicating.
- Speak clearly and a little slower than usual.
- Smile.
- Use your name when you start to speak.
- Use their name.
- Move calmly.
- Show pictures or objects when asking the person to make choices if they cannot understand the spoken word easily.
- Follow their lead in the conversation.

Do not:

- Stress the person (this is perhaps the most important thing to remember).
- Contradict the person. If they think that they are 40 years younger than they are, then they may well not know who you are or even if they have been married and had children.
- Raise your voice.
- Talk fast.
- Talk metaphorically, e.g. 'It's raining cats and dogs.'
- Ask questions if they are going to struggle answering them. Asking what they did over the weekend, for example, may panic them if they cannot remember.
- Rush the person.

To return to the story of Jane at the beginning of this chapter, you can now see how Jane's response contradicted Sally's reality and caused her stress and grief. The best response would have been to smile and go along with Sally's reality. Once she started to sing again she would have returned to the present activity.

This chapter has provided a very brief overview of dementia and its effect on people with the condition. There is a list at the end of the book of books which will provide much more information.

PART TWO

Preparing to Get Started

It is essential that you and all others involved are well prepared and knowledgeable about the various aspects of running singing sessions. You will learn much as you go along, but if you are not well prepared from the beginning there is a good chance that people will not continue to come, you will feel frustrated and disappointed and, of course, a great activity will have been lost.

There are, of course, some significant differences between setting up a group in a residential home and setting up a group in a wider community. Where pertinent these differences will be highlighted.

Before preparing individual sessions in detail there are a number of things that need to be addressed to make sure you are well prepared. They are:

- Preparing yourself.

- Preparing others.

- Being clear about the roles of people involved.

- Identifying a suitable venue.

- Letting people know about your group.

- Having a committee and constitution (if appropriate).

CHAPTER FOUR

Preparing yourself

As stated at the very beginning of this book, it is not essential that you are an accomplished musician. It will help, but what is more important is that you have the enthusiasm and drive to galvanise others into being part of a team.

If this is all new to you, then find out as much as you can about other singing groups. You could contact your local Alzheimer's society and ask if they have a 'Singing for the Brain' group that you could attend. This is not to suggest that you run your group as they do, but you will get some good ideas.

There may well be other groups running already in your community, so try to find them. The group that I am involved in has had many visitors who have then gone off to set up their own groups. Do not be shy of asking if you can attend for a few sessions.

There may also be a group running in a local home for older people, and the regulatory body charged with inspecting homes in your area should be able to tell you which homes already run singing groups.

If you are going to be one of the people leading the singing, it might be worth your while finding a singing teacher to give you some information about exercises you can do for your voice and especially to help you project your voice. This is not essential but may give you a bit more confidence. Many people will, however, be perfectly able to lead the singing without this extra help.

Get some friends together and run a singing group with them and get their feedback on how you do. If you are working in a home for older people, get some of the staff together for a session . . . be brave!

Hopefully this book will equip you with most of what you need to know.

CHAPTER FIVE

Preparing others

The first thing is to determine who these 'others' might be. They may well include staff, family, friends and volunteers.

Whether you are running your group in a residential home, in a nursing home, in a sheltered housing complex or in the community, there will be many common aspects required of the people helping with the running of the group. There are, however, some differences. For this reason the settings will be covered separately.

Residential homes, nursing homes and day care facilities

Staff

If setting up a group in a residential home, nursing home or day care facility, you will need to involve other staff. It is very important that the singing group does not become a place where people are left without members of staff being involved. The singing needs to be seen as an integral part of the home or the activities of the centre, and all, or at least most, staff need to be involved at some level. This does not mean they have to actually take part in the group, but they need to know about it, know why it is running, know when it is running and know what their role is in helping people to attend the group.

You should involve the manager as much as possible. Often what happens is that someone sets up a singing group in a home and it becomes that person's 'baby' or 'project'. When they leave the group dwindles or stops. The group must be incorporated into the fabric of the home. Hopefully it is not an add-on that the activities coordinator runs alone but is a joint effort with as many staff involved as possible.

In a later chapter there is information about committees and constitutions. This really applies, if at all, to community groups. In a residential setting a committee and constitution will not be necessary but it is useful to have at least a small group of people to help with the various tasks involved. They do not have to be a 'committee' but they do need to identify with the singing group.

You will need to make sure that there are sufficient staff in each session to support the residents. This is particularly important if you have songs that you walk or dance to.

It can be quite hard to get staff involved in singing groups. There are a number of reasons for this. I list below reasons that I have been given.

- Shyness.
- 'I am not musical.'
- 'Not my job.'
- 'I am rushed off my feet already.'
- Other staff seeing it as a soft option and making comments such as 'Have you enjoyed your rest, then?'

There need to be a number of responses to this. Certainly I would not dismiss the fact that staff often feel under a lot of pressure. Staffing levels in some homes are woefully low and pared to the minimum. However, providing leisure and pleasure to residents is not just the remit of the activities coordinator. It is certainly not an add-on. Leisure and pleasure need to be seen as integral to the holistic care and support of everyone, and this means that staff are to be involved.

Some people will be hesitant about taking on a new activity and may be shy about singing, but with encouragement my experience is they usually enjoy it once they get over their anxiety.

It is also important to emphasise that staff do not have to be especially musical but just able to hold a tune.

Family and friends

The other group of people you should consider involving is people's family and friends.

Mary

Mary had been visiting her mother for five months since her admission to a residential care home. Mary found the visits stressful and was increasingly reluctant to visit. This was because when she was with her mother it was very hard to sustain any sort of conversation; in fact at times her mother did not even recognise Mary as her daughter.

When the activities coordinator started a singing group she asked Mary and other relatives if they wanted to come along.

This was a turning point in Mary's involvement with her mother and indeed with the home generally.

Mary was able to sing along with her mother, who sang songs with joy and recognition. Some of the songs were ones she had sung to Mary as a child and this was particularly poignant.

Mary now had a focus for her time with her mother, but also it was a focus that was often joyful and had meaning for them both.

Mary also got to know other residents in the group and the other staff who were also involved.

This story is not so unusual. Involving family in singing groups is a great way to enable them to be involved and maintain some communication.

Getting a wide group of people involved in the singing group

One way to get people involved is to have an 'open day' type of event. One home I know of held an event for residents, tenants, family, friends, staff and volunteers. Adverts were put up within the home and in the community. Leaflets were given to visitors and management were asked to arrange cover for any staff who wanted to attend. Refreshments were provided, a talk was given on the benefits of singing and then a short singing session was held just to illustrate the point.

**Caroline House
Caroline Bank Avenue**

A music club is being set up at the above address. An open day will take place between 10.30am and 2.00pm on Friday 28th November.

 Morning refreshments will be served from 10.30am

11.30am Concert and sing-along ('Getting to Know You')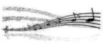

12.30pm Pre-lunch sherry

1.00pm Buffet lunch

The music club will provide support and entertainment for sheltered housing tenants and residential home residents, and would welcome anyone in the community who would like to join in to sing along or be entertained.

There will be time for discussion on how to develop the group, timing, frequency, volunteering, programme content, song requests and involvement with the running of the group. We will also be looking for people interested in organising fundraising events to support the running of the club.

Please phone number 00001111111 Monday–Friday between 10.00am and 4.30pm to reserve a place.

This advert resulted in a group being run on a regular basis with family, friends, volunteers and service users being involved. The group ran for many years before a change of management closed it down.

In the community, including 'sheltered housing' type facilities

If you are running a group in the community then you will need to give serious thought to whether you have people's family, friends or paid carers in attendance. There are a number of things to take into account. Not least are the needs of the carer.

John

John, whose wife had dementia, attended the group for two years. During that time he said he found the support of other carers in an informal setting invaluable. He was able to talk to others going through similar difficulties, but it was done in a relaxed social environment. He felt valued by others just when, because of his commitments to his wife and because friends found the situation hard to face, his old social network was breaking down.

John also found the singing cheered him up and gave him a 'happy feeling'.

The session provided him with an opportunity to enjoy his wife's joy, something that happened less and less in their lives.

Carers attending singing groups speak of the benefits that they gain from being with their partner. Sometimes this is beyond simply doing something together; the session can provide an opportunity for something deeper.

I have also noticed that sometimes the song will enable the carer to sing words to their partner that they want to express but cannot in the spoken word. 'You Made Me Love You' and 'If You Were the Only Girl in the World' are two that have brought a tear to the eye.

Adult protection issues

There is legislation in the UK designed to protect vulnerable adults. This legislation requires that everyone working with vulnerable adults, and this includes people with dementia, must have a police check carried out.

In the residential and day care setting there will be staff who have had their police checks done and who are qualified and able to care for people's needs, including intimate things such as helping people to use the toilet.

In the community, if people come without a carer, then the people running the group are responsible. Under the 'protection of vulnerable adults' legislation all volunteers would need to have police checks carried out. Volunteers would also have to be competent to provide the care people might need. Some of the group might need personal care. There would also be a need for a large number of volunteers in order to be sufficiently able to watch and monitor everyone.

Pamela

Pamela had been attending the singing group for a year. She was always accompanied by either her sister or a paid carer.

On one occasion she turned up without her sister. She was allowed to stay as she had made such an effort to attend. There was an anticipation that maybe her sister would turn up. This did not happen, but Pamela was fully engaged with the events of the afternoon.

At the end of the session everyone was busy leaving when it was noticed that Pamela had left. Her coat, hat, scarf and gloves were still on her chair. It was a freezing winter's day outside, sleet and snow with a biting north-westerly wind.

This incident served to highlight the vulnerability of some participants and the need for either a carer to accompany every person with dementia or for an increased number of suitably competent and checked volunteers.

Volunteers

Another group of people who you may want to involve is volunteers. In a home this might not be so necessary, but if you do use volunteers then you will need to carry out police checks as detailed above. If you are running a group in the community then probably the volunteers will be essential.

First get your volunteers. This is not necessarily an easy process. We, and indeed other people I know from other groups, have found that to start the best way is to use people known to the organisers. This often means that the volunteer group will have a particular character. So one group has a lot of ex-social-workers, another group has predominantly ex-teachers, and another mostly musicians. Many towns and cities will have organisations that help put you in touch with volunteers. It is important, however, that you have clear ideas about the qualities and skills that you are looking for.

Judy

> Judy was recently retired and widowed. She was lonely and desperate for company. Her mother had had dementia and Judy felt confident that she would know what was wanted in a singing group for people with dementia.
>
> Judy volunteered to serve tea and coffee and to talk to people.
>
> Despite training on dementia and the needs of people with dementia, Judy talked constantly about herself and her mother during group sessions. Clearly the sessions were acting as a form of therapy for her. She enjoyed the social contact but was not sensitive to the needs of people with dementia and their carers.
>
> An attempt was made to give her work in the kitchen preparing the tea and coffee, but she constantly left this to talk 'at' others.
>
> The organisers had to find a way of suggesting that this was not an appropriate group for Judy.

It is important to be aware of the potential conflict of interest between the volunteers' needs and those of people with dementia. Some of this can be circumvented by providing volunteers with good information and training (Chapter Three, 'What do you need to know about dementia?' should provide useful information for everyone involved).

You also need to be clear about the different tasks that you may require of volunteers so that you can match their skills and interests to your requirements.

It is also important to recognise that people volunteer because they want to be useful and contribute. If people are not allocated tasks they can feel redundant and not valued and they may leave.

CHAPTER SIX

Roles of people involved

Depending on your role and the setting, the following are some of the key roles you may need. Some may be carried out by volunteers, some by paid staff.

The singing leader

You need someone to lead the singing. It may be possible to run with one person doing this. My experience, however, is that it is better to have more than one person to allow for holidays, sickness etc. This also means that there are different styles and often different songs depending on the leader, and this adds to the variety and mix.

The qualities required of the singing leader are more than just the ability to sing. In fact, so long as the leader can hold a tune, there are other attributes that are just as, if not more, important and need to be present. The following may appear daunting but many people do possess these qualities or can develop them.

The leader has to be confident in speaking to and directing a room full of people, many of whom may be strangers (to the leader and each other) at first.

The leader must be able to engage with the whole group with enthusiasm and self-confidence (although initially you may have to fake this if you are nervous). Of course the leader needs to smile and make lots of eye contact with the participants.

By watching the group closely the leader should be able to gauge how things are going. You may find that some songs are not working but others go down well, which may mean adjusting the programme as you go along. If people enjoy a song, sing it again; if not, make a note not to include it again. If some people are looking distressed or not engaged, try to sing to them and SMILE.

Remember to slow your speech down a bit and project your voice when talking so that everyone can easily hear you.

Do not talk fast and do not talk for long. It is good to make links between songs and even to tell little anecdotes, but do not be long-winded. Watch to see if people are following you.

Do not stand behind anything or, indeed, stand still; move into the group and engage.

Remember that people with dementia will be looking for visual cues as verbal information is becoming harder to follow, so use your body and facial expression to convey things whenever possible.

The accompanist

It may be that you will not have an accompanist. An accompanist is not at all essential, but it does make life easier if you have an instrument to provide a strong beat to the group and to give you backing and keep the tune.

If you do have an accompanist it is very useful to have people who can 'busk' and not be completely dependent on the musical score. Such people are like gold dust, so do not worry if this is not possible; do not be put off. Even playing the tune in the right hand will be a help to rhythm and pitch.

Keyboard accompaniment is perhaps the most suitable. An electric keyboard or electric piano can alter the key when necessary and provide accompanying chords, but you could also use a guitar, if the group is not too big, or indeed any other instrument if it can be heard above the singing.

Sometimes the accompanist needs to be able to alter the key of songs. Many keyboards will do this for you, so do not worry too much about this.

Just as with the leader, the accompanist needs to be engaged and SMILE.

Hospitality providers

You will also need people to make and serve refreshments.

If you are running your group in a residential home/day care setting this might not be an extra task as participants may already have had their tea or lunch. However, it can be a good thing to introduce as part of the session to facilitate the social interaction between everyone before you start the singing. It can make it more of an occasion and separate it from usual daily routine.

Sherry

> Sherry with cake provided a wonderful atmosphere of afternoons out and entertainment in one home.
>
> All the participants were offered a seat and some sherry or a non-alcoholic soft drink which they consumed with small cakes and biscuits before the singing began.
>
> This gave the afternoon events a nice warm feeling of being a bit special and celebratory.

In the community, people who make the tea need to arrive early and have everything sorted and ready. Once the participants start to arrive they need to be quick off the mark providing refreshments. People with dementia will not necessarily understand why they are at a table if no drinks or food arrive. (More detail is given about what needs to be in place in part three.)

The people providing hospitality need to know how to communicate with people with dementia; for example, asking them to make choices between various drinks might be too confusing. Show choices rather than asking questions.

People with dementia

The most important people involved are, of course, the people with dementia. Their participation is central. They are not passive recipients of entertainment but are the providers of the singing and the culture of the group. The role of the participants is something that needs to be constantly attended to. If this is not emphasised sufficiently then the group can become dominated by the needs of the staff and volunteers.

Whilst the group is for people with dementia, this does not mean it is for all people with dementia.

Sometimes a delicate situation occurs when a resident cannot cope with the dynamics of the singing group and that person can become disruptive. Often the disruption is caused by the resident constantly calling out inappropriately. The singing group is frequently interrupted to attend to their needs.

This has to be addressed to enable the singing group to continue and to prevent other residents becoming disturbed and distressed. If other residents become uneasy with the situation they will eventually decline the invitation to attend as their enjoyment has ceased.

In situations like this there is a need to look at how staff can support the resident who is disruptive in the group setting and see how their need for musical involvement can be met. This may be by using one-to-one sessions where staff can work with music and song that suits the pace and musical taste of the individual.

I came across the following situation in one home.

A singing group had been running for two months in the lounge of a residential home. Fifteen people attended regularly and thoroughly enjoyed the experience.

A new resident was encouraged to attend. This woman was extremely agitated. She screamed and swore loudly throughout the session. The singing did not calm her.

This had a very disturbing effect on the other residents.

The singing leader asked staff not to bring the new lady to the group. She, the leader, was told that the woman would continue to come as it was as much her right to be there as anyone else's.

Clearly no one was enjoying the situation. For everyone's benefit the lady needed to be elsewhere. She would have probably been much better served if she had had one-to-one attention. I think that there was also a feeling that the singing group had become a 'dumping ground' and the staff were leaving the lady there rather than attending to her specific needs. Hopefully this is an uncommon situation.

CHAPTER SEVEN

Identifying a suitable venue

In a residential/nursing home and some sheltered housing and day centres

If you are providing the sessions within a residential setting it may be that you have a choice of the lounge or the dining room. The problem with using the lounge is that other residents may well be there or wanting to use it. The dining room is usually not as cosy and there may be problems with the furniture if you intend to use activities such as walking or dancing to some songs. People with dementia will not want to be in a room that feels crowded or is too noisy (singing in the dining room may be too loud and echoing).

It is preferable to find a separate space for the singing.

Most homes nowadays will have more than one lounge. You will need to identify one for the group and make sure that it is reserved on a regular basis. Prior to the group meeting reserve the room and put a sign on the door saying that the music group will be meeting, stating start and finish times. If the room is not accessible in sufficient time to prepare it or, even worse, if it has been double-booked, the singing group will not be a calm or predictable event.

The room needs to be well lit with chairs preferably arranged in a horseshoe if possible. You need to make sure the leader can see everyone clearly, and everyone needs to be able to see the leader. Take account of the various difficulties some people may have. Make sure that there is sufficient space for staff, family and volunteers to be interspersed with the residents. This will be especially important for residents who may become agitated or start to shout or behave in ways that may be upsetting to others. It is important that people who behave in this way are not automatically excluded but that staff try to be beside them and act as a calming presence.

A further consideration is to make sure that the area outside the room is not noisy. It can be disturbing for the people in the group if there is noise that they cannot control or make sense of. I have been to groups where the staff have been talking, shouting and even vacuuming outside or near the room. This is, of course, a reason for the singing group to be integrated into the home's daily routine, for all staff, including domestic workers, to know about the group, and for the manager to make sure that tasks that are noisy are not carried out near the room where the singing is taking place.

Picking a venue in the community

This can be tricky. Care homes and day care settings already have premises, equipment to make and serve refreshments, and possibly a keyboard and projector. In the community it is more complicated and requires more planning and research.

It is a matter not just of finding a place but of getting a place that is available when you want it. Certainly people will often find this a bit of a hurdle. It is worthwhile checking out church halls which may be standing empty; the church might offer the hall free of charge. I know of one group with access to a delightful room in a hotel that does not charge anything but sees the benefits in terms of the community and people coming to the hotel at other times.

When choosing a venue the following things need to be taken into consideration:

- You need to think about the times that would be best for the people coming to the group. Too late in the afternoon and people will be tired and maybe more confused. The morning may put the carer under pressure to get everything ready to come.
- Access is an issue. Remember that people with dementia can have problems with steps because of their difficulties judging distance and depth. This may also be the case with patterned carpets where the different colours can look as if they are holes or steps.
- You need to check on public transport. How easy will it be for people to get to you and return home?

- Parking facilities are also very important. People will not want to walk far from their car.
- Toilets must be accessible.
- Access to a kitchen for preparing drinks.
- Check heating and lighting. There needs to be a good heat source that can be put on long before the session in cool weather. People cannot sit in a cool room. Lighting needs to be good; some people will have problems with seeing and dull light will exacerbate their problems.
- Check if there is a cost for using the venue, how much this is and what it covers. If there is rent to be paid for the premises and equipment to purchase, then consideration should be given to fundraising.
- Public liability insurance is worth considering for any group. The group will not be automatically covered by the premises' public liability insurance.

CHAPTER EIGHT

Fundraising

It may be that, initially, a group starts on a shoestring, borrowing equipment etc. Do not let lack of substantial funds put you off. My experience is that, once you start, people will start to give money.

- Some groups charge a small fee of around £1 for participants. This does help towards the cost of refreshments. It is perhaps just as effective to have donation tins on tables. This means that people feel free to come even if they have no money or have forgotten to bring any. Supermarkets are good at providing refreshment supplies ... just ask.
- Some supermarkets run schemes where customers deposit tokens in boxes in support of local charities and associations. Depending on the number of tokens deposited, each charity/association will receive money. This is always well worth the while.
- Supermarkets that charge a 5p fee for plastic bags have to give the money to charity. Why not yours?
- Having bring-and-buy afternoon teas can raise substantial amounts.
- Apply for grants from local authorities or local benevolent societies. The internet should find local organisations that provide grants.
- Local businesses, such as banks, law firms etc., often give money. Many businesses have a policy to support a charity. Ask as many businesses as you can and at least one will come up trumps.

CHAPTER NINE

Letting people know about your group

In a residential home

If you are setting up a group in a residential home, you will have a slightly different task to a community group. Obviously to start with you know the population that you will be drawing your participants from. You will have an idea about who would benefit most from the group. I would, however, caution against any decisions about suitability. As described in Chapter One, everyone benefits from music and responds to it. The issue for the person setting up the group is more about whether some people might find the group too crowding and busy and the noise of all the singing too loud. For such people singing on a one-to-one basis should be considered; do not deprive people of music because they cannot manage a group.

You should advertise the group in various places around the home and in the home newsletter, if there is one, and talk to people about their interest in music and being part of the group.

Poster for home

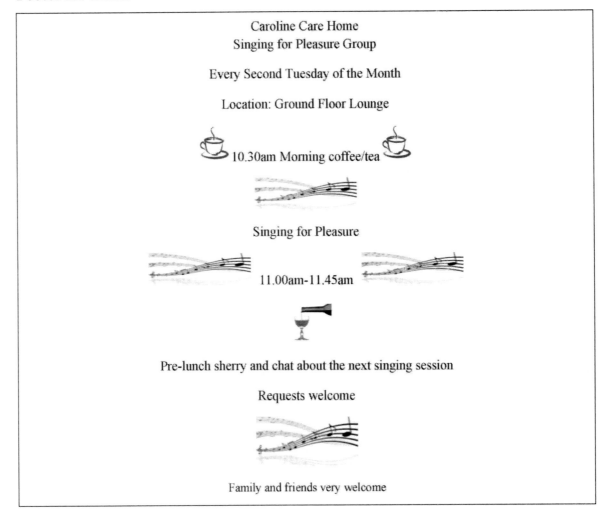

Caroline Care Home
Singing for Pleasure Group

Every Second Tuesday of the Month

Location: Ground Floor Lounge

10.30am Morning coffee/tea

Singing for Pleasure

11.00am-11.45am

Pre-lunch sherry and chat about the next singing session

Requests welcome

Family and friends very welcome

In the community

If you are starting a group in the community then you have a much harder task on your hands. You need to advertise in places such as:

- Doctors' surgeries.
- The memory clinic if there is one.

- The local branch of the Alzheimer's society.
- Local shops and supermarkets.
- Churches.
- Day services for older people.
- Carers' groups.
- Hospitals.
- Social work departments.
- Local papers and community newsletters.
- You might even try to get a slot on the local radio to talk about the group.

Produce a leaflet giving information. The following is one that we have used for a number of groups. Feel free to adapt it to your group.

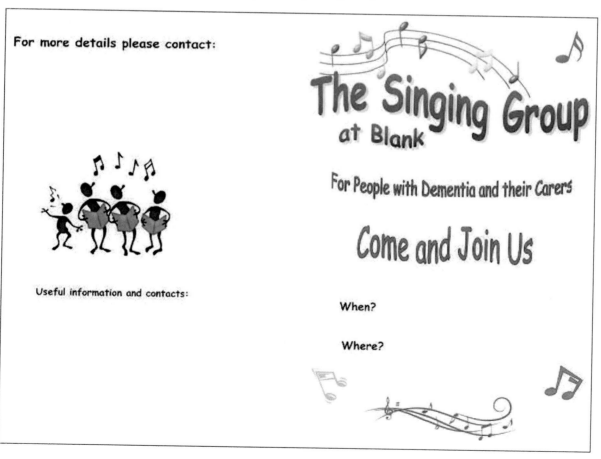

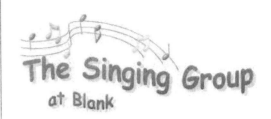

The Singing Group
at Blank

Who is this group for?

It is for people with Dementia who enjoy singing and who are still able to live at home in the community. The group also provides support for their carer(s).

Who are we?

We are an independent group that provides opportunities for people with Dementia and their carer(s) to come together **to socialise and to sing**, with the emphasis on **enjoyment and fun**. We are not a choir, and do not aim for performances.

What happens?

We meet for coffee and a chat first, giving people a chance to socialise and also to find help, advice or support from volunteers or other members of the group. After that, **we sing together** enjoyably and in a relaxed atmosphere for around 45 minutes. There is a singing leader and an accompanist. Our repertoire is varied and is built upon requests from members. Songs include favourites from yesteryear, songs from musicals and films, and some rounds.

Often there is a simple music quiz, and each session includes a selection of Scottish songs as these are very popular. We sit in a circle to allow everyone to feel equal and not indentified by their illness. This helps to promote feelings of belonging.

The Sessions give participants a positive view of life. The lively atmosphere encourages communication and helps to relieve the tension and isolation that illnesses such as Dementia can bring about. These benefits, experienced by all, often extend beyond the sessions as people return home.

What are our aims?

The Singing Group offers stimulating and social activities designed to enhance well-being, and provide enjoyment and confidence to lives affected by memory problems and Dementia. Research shows that such activity reduces stress and agitation – encouraging a 'feel good' factor in all.

Volunteers are on hand but those with dementia should be accompanied. There is no charge, but a small donation towards refreshments is appreciated.

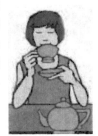

CHAPTER TEN

Having a committee and a constitution

The committee

This might not seem to be particularly important in a residential setting, and indeed in most settings groups operate without committee or constitution. The danger of not having a committee or at least some specified group of people is that the ownership and organisation of the singing group falls to one person, usually the activities coordinator or someone who has agreed to come in and run the group. This means that there is no general involvement in the organisation and running of the group, it is seen as an 'add-on' and if the individual responsible leaves or is ill the group is at risk.

Community groups will need much more coordination; as well as managing a team of volunteers, they will need to identify appropriate premises and negotiate terms, borrow or purchase equipment and fundraise.

The committee will need to identify the members with strong organisation skills who will organise all the practical elements of the group behind the scenes and on the day.

It is important that the group does not become too big and bureaucratic. Try to have about four people involved in a committee. In a residential setting, if one of these were to be the manager of the home, that would be an excellent way of maintaining continuity and organisational commitment.

In the community you are very likely to need some sort of committee. You will need people to carry out tasks such as:

- Publicity.
- Hiring space.
- Advertising.

- Recruiting and managing volunteers.
- Keeping a music library.
- Fundraising.
- Organising special events.
- Managing the money.

The constitution

In a residential setting this will not be necessary, although it is a good idea to have some ground rules written down.

In the community it really is much more important to have a constitution. This probably feels rather formal and daunting, but if you are running any group in the community which involves a large group of people it is very important to be clear about your aims, rules and financial management. It will be essential to have a constitution if you want to register as a charity.

What you do not want is to get caught up in lots of formal things when all you want to do is run a singing group. To facilitate your drawing-up of a constitution a sample is included in the appendix.

PART THREE

Planning, Organising and Running Sessions

This section is designed to help you plan, organise and run sessions. It will detail the structure of the sessions, with reasons for using different types of songs and singing arrangements. These are, of course, only guides and each group will need to adapt according to the needs of the participants, the skills of the volunteers and staff, the time available and the support given.

CHAPTER ELEVEN

Practical organisation of the sessions

Before the singing starts there are other organisational considerations. Some of these apply more to community settings than to residential settings but some are relevant to both.

Remember in all the practical arrangements you need to be constantly aware of the need to strive to provide a warm, welcoming, calm and safe environment.

Refreshments: If refreshments are being served, tables and chairs will need to be put in place and tables set with cups, milk, sugar and biscuits. Space around the tables is important, bearing in mind that there could be wheelchair users and frail older people with mobility problems.

In residential settings it may be necessary to arrange for the kitchen staff to provide a trolley of refreshments specifically for the group. It should be in the room before people arrive. You do not want the group to be disturbed by the regular refreshments trolley being wheeled in during the session.

If there is to be no charge for the group it is an idea to place 'donation tins' on the tables and allow members to donate towards their tea/coffee

Music playing on arrival: This could be a CD playing or someone playing an instrument. (This gets drowned out when things get busy.)

Meeting and greeting: In the community a great emphasis should be put on welcoming people as they walk in the door and directing or accompanying them towards the registration point and/or the tables for refreshments.

In residential settings it is important that people who are brought to the session are attended to whilst they find a seat and settle in. I have seen staff simply bring people and leave them; this has led to people becoming agitated as they can feel abandoned and unsure of what they are meant to be doing.

Registration: In the community, members and volunteers need to register in case of fire. Name badges should be considered as remembering the names of a large group of people is tricky for everyone. These can be issued at registration.

Socialising and participation: Volunteers should sit at tables while refreshments are being served, facilitating conversation, introducing members to each other and giving particular attention to new members. They should also sit with members during the singing and encourage members to participate. Volunteers should be safety-conscious if walking round with members who are frail, although carers are ultimately responsible for the person with dementia.

CHAPTER TWELVE

Various session formats

An important consideration is the length of the session. You will need to decide how long suits the participants, taking into account any other commitments they have. How much energy do you have? Will people have refreshments first? If so, how long will that leave for the rest of the session? This may be an issue in residential homes where meals may be at set times. In the community you may need to think about people getting home, especially in the winter when it gets dark earlier.

Below are examples of differently structured, timed and presented sessions. Each one is catering for a different group of people with different needs in different settings. They are given to illustrate the fact that there is no single way to run a session. You can see from just these examples how different settings with different needs amongst the participants can lead to some notable differences in the way sessions are timed and run.

Two residential homes

Timing

In Home A the group is run in the mornings as this is the time when people with dementia are likely to be at their most alert. The session lasts for one and a half hours with tea and coffee at the beginning. At the end of the session sherry is served as an aperitif before people go off to lunch.

In Home B the group is run in the afternoon between 1.45 and 2.45. This is because the activities coordinator has found that for many residents the afternoon drags and people want some activity. Many people are a bit sleepy after lunch but the music seems to revive them.

Attendance

Both homes have up to 20 people with dementia attending the group. In Home A there are eight helpers who include members of staff, volunteers and family members.

In Home B the aim is to have a minimum of three people: the activities coordinator and the two volunteer leaders who run the sessions. Sometimes there is also the chaplain, a domestic and another member of staff. Occasionally there is a pianist to accompany the songs. When this is not possible, people sing unaccompanied. Very well-known songs are sung at such times.

In this home CDs are often used for a few of the songs when there is not an accompanist.

Typical songs from one programme

Up to 20 songs are sung. These are a combination of songs decided in advance by the leader and ones that emerge from the group during the session. The songs cover a wide range but there is a predominance of songs from musicals, wartime songs and popular songs of the fifties.

A community group for people with early onset dementia

Timing

This group is for younger people with dementia. It runs in the evenings from seven to eight o'clock because people's carers are still going to work and are not always free in the day to accompany their husband/wife to the group. The use of volunteers or paid carers might facilitate daytime sessions but people would often rather come with their partner.

Attendance

There might only be five people with dementia attending with their carers. This is a much smaller group than most. The smallness of the group allows for an intimacy and individual response not so easily achieved in the bigger groups.

The group does have a pianist to accompany the singing, but this is not always the case. With such a small group it is perhaps easier to sing without the benefit of a piano, although it is a great support to the fewer voices.

Typical songs from one programme

These are a little different from the songs sung with the older people's groups. The age range of people in the early onset group is younger and so more recent songs are often chosen. Whilst there are songs from the fifties there are also songs from the sixties and seventies, reflecting the different age of many of the people in this group

A community group for older people with dementia and their carers

Timing

This group is run in the afternoons. This is because carers (husbands, wives, friends or paid carers) will need to get the person with dementia ready and take them to the singing group. This is often too much of a rush in the morning. Holding the group after lunch means that the carer has had time to prepare and also it provides an activity for the afternoon, which can drag out if nothing is provided.

Attendance

There can be an issue about the number of attendees. This can be more unpredictable in the community, where things like bad weather, holidays and family commitments can have an effect. One of the groups I have been involved in had 80 people turn up one afternoon; this included volunteers and family carers. Apart from being an indication of the great need for such a group, it was also a fire risk and made the group too big for people with dementia.

This group has a piano accompanist.

Typical songs from one programme

Songs for this group include music hall favourites, songs from both world wars, songs from most of the best-known musicals, well-known songs from the fifties and early sixties.

The brief overview above is an indication of how varied groups can be.

It is worth noting that the size of the group will have an effect on the way in which the group is run. With a large group the leaders need to be more prescriptive and have a well-structured programme. This does mean that a degree of spontaneity is lost, but requests should be accommodated where possible. With smaller groups it is easier to be more responsive to any requests. It is also easier to have conversations between songs. In a large group, if the leader has a conversation with someone then a large number of people will not be able to follow and will feel left out.

CHAPTER THIRTEEN

Helping with the words

It is important to emphasise that getting the words right is not a primary focus. I always say that it is just as good to sing 'la di da di da'. I do sometimes sing 'la di da di da' to emphasise this point. It is important that the participants do not feel under any pressure to 'get it right'. Some people may just whistle if they cannot vocalise.

Song sheets can be a useful and successful guide to the singing. Most people would use them for choirs, carol singing etc. They do, however, present problems for many older people and particularly for people with dementia. I have, mostly, found song sheets more unhelpful than helpful. They can be distracting for various reasons:

- People may be unable to follow the line of words.
- Problems with dexterity may make turning or even holding pages difficult.
- People may have problems with concentration.
- Sheets are dropped on the floor.
- People will spend time flicking through the pages.
- People will be looking down at the song sheet rather than up at the leader or other people in the group.

Song sheets can become something that highlights the losses associated with dementia, failing eyesight and loss of manual dexterity.

Song sheets can be used more discriminately by handing out a sheet for a specific song rather than handing out sheets for an entire session; this removes the problems with handling lots of paper. It also means that the person without dementia could hold the sheet, if necessary, and then hand it back or put it under the chair once the song is over.

Another option is to staple sheets together in the order in which you are going to sing. This does not get over all the problems but does reduce the likelihood of things being dropped on the floor.

One option is to throw out the words verbally first, to trigger or lead into lines of the lyrics. This does not have to be every line, sometimes just the first line of the verse or chorus depending on the song. This is an old-fashioned and well-tested technique used in music hall and variety. It gives an extra oomph to the sessions.

Projecting words onto a screen can be effective. This means that people are looking up and to the front of the group. It also means that the words can be shown in small sections to avoid presenting too much information for participants to cope with. A disadvantage of this is that the words need to be loaded onto a PowerPoint presentation before each session. Moreover, the leader has to keep remembering to click the mouse to change the words, or there has to be another person available to do this. It also means that there is a piece of equipment in the room that people need to be careful of, especially when walking or dancing to songs.

Most songs will still be under copyright; the copyright only falls 70 years after the composer's death. To get the necessary permission to use copyrighted material you will need to contact the Performing Rights Society. There will be an annual fee for this.

CHAPTER FOURTEEN

Structuring a programme

It is important that you plan and structure sessions rather than choose the songs 'en route' or 'ad hoc' as you will need to ensure appropriateness, familiarity, variety and timing. It is also particularly helpful for people with dementia to have a familiar formula and routine. The occasional spontaneous song can be fun and work well if the leader is familiar with it and confident, but this should be in the context of a well-prepared session.

Below is a general outline structure. It is given as a template only. The following chapters will expand on the various points made here and will provide detailed information.

Structuring the session

1. Introduce yourself and anyone else involved in leading the session such as the pianist and, if you have one, the projectionist. Give a clap.
2. Welcome everyone. If there are new people, acknowledge them in a general way: 'There are some new people here today, so welcome, and I hope you enjoy yourself.' Smile!
3. Reiterate that the point of the session is to enjoy yourself and not to worry if you do not know the words; just sing 'la di da di da'. Some people may not be able to do this either but may whistle.
4. Warm-up exercises – to prepare the group for the session.
5. Sing a song to open the session. It is a good idea to have the same one every time.
6. After a few songs sung sitting down and in unison, begin to introduce variety. Start to intersperse songs to walk/dance to, rounds, partner songs, call-and-response songs and songs divided between men and women.
7. Have a short and entertaining musical quiz.

8. Towards the end of the session sing calmer songs.

9. Sing a closing song. It is a good idea to have the same song every time. Use a song that has 'goodbye' in it and wave. In a residential home where people are not going to be leaving, this might not be a good idea. A song such as 'Here's to the Next Time' would be more appropriate.

10. Go round and sing 'goodbye' to everyone.

CHAPTER FIFTEEN

Choosing warm-up exercises

There are many different ways to warm up. Your choice will depend on the participants' abilities and needs and your capacity for making things up. Remember to engender as much laughter as you can and find a happy medium between spending too long on the warm-ups and rushing to get on with the singing. My experience is that generally not enough time is spent on the warm-ups.

Below are some suggestions that you could develop to suit your group. None of these require you to be a choirmaster or very musical. They are just ways of getting the body and mind ready to have a good hearty sing-song.

You will see from Chapter Three, 'What do you need to know about dementia?', that people will often have problems engaging in purposeful movements. This means that even apparently simple things like clapping hands or raising arms or shoulders may be difficult. When doing warm-up exercises, watch the group, and if people are struggling with a particular exercise then abandon it. Exercises using the legs may be a problem for people in wheelchairs, so suggest, perhaps, that they tap their thighs instead.

Some tried and tested warm-ups

Below is a list of warm-up exercises that work well with people with dementia who may have problems with coordinating their body movements. They are also suitable for people who are sitting down close to others.

It is a good idea to do the full range of these exercises before a session, but this may not always be suitable. It may be that people who have come to sing do not fully understand why they need to do these exercises or they may find them embarrassing to do. I once had a lady in a group express some bewilderment. She thought she had come to a keep-fit class by mistake. It is important that the leader explains, simply, that the purpose of the exercises is to get people's voices, lungs and bodies ready for a good singing session. Try to engender some amusement in the warm-ups.

Shoulders	Lift shoulders, breathing in, then relax them, breathing out. Do this four times.	Begins to relax the upper body.
Hands	Wring hands as if they are being washed. Then shake them dry.	Begins to take tension out of the hands and shoulders.
Breathing	Lift arms up in front parallel with shoulders. Take a deep breath, then, breathing out and lowering arms, say 'he'. Repeat with 'ho', then 'ha'. Depending on the group, do each of these between one and three times.	Begins to help people concentrate on breathing. It is also the first sound they are making together and if you can get a laugh this will further relax people.
Breathing	Now put hands on your tummy. Take a deep breath in. Breathing out, repeat 'he he he', 'ha ha ha' and 'ho ho ho' and feel the tummy moving. Depending on the group, do these between one and three times.	Can enable deeper breathing.
The mouth and making a sound	Remind people of when they were young and chewed bubble gum. Get them to chew as if they had bubble gum. Then remind them how we used to pull the gum out of our mouths and suck it back. Using a hand pretend to pull gum out and up. As you do, sing a rising note. Then push it back in using a descending note. This will make people laugh.	Now people will be making a note together; this will help people relax, laugh and begin to smile, often at each other. This will all help people to come out of themselves if they are anxious.
Legs	Do a light step in place about ten times, and then build up quickly to a loud stomp, with arms now moving as if you are marching.	This will loosen up the lower body as well as the arms. If people are in wheelchairs and cannot raise their legs then they can just tap their thighs.
Breathing and stretching	Stretch and yawn as if you have just got up.	This will further relax people. People will also make quite a noise and this usually engenders laughter.

CHAPTER SIXTEEN

Choosing songs: what, why and how?

When choosing songs it is important to remember that as we age our voices get lower, so many songs are written too high for older people. The second D above middle C is probably as high as you should expect people to sing. Either choose songs that are low enough or transpose songs down a bit. This may sound daunting to those people not knowledgeable about music, but if you have a pianist they will know what to do. The best thing is to have an electric piano or keyboard which has a transpose button! If you are singing unaccompanied, just remember to sing down below the upper D.

It is, however, important not to have all your songs in the same key and pitch as this is not good for the voice or mood. A good variety is what you are looking for.

If, as is the case for some groups, you use CDs as backing to accompany the singing, you need to make sure that the songs are not pitched too high. Max Bygraves sings most of his songs in an easy key. They are also good songs to sing along to. Certainly I know groups that love and know his repertoire.

The disadvantage of using recorded music is that it is unforgiving. If people sing more slowly or otherwise change the tempo, the track will not accommodate this as would be the case with a live accompanist.

The music used will be a combination of tunes the leaders have chosen and requests from the group. It is important that the choice of songs reflects the preferences of the participants. Leaders may well have favourites, but these may not be shared by the participants. In one group I heard of the leader was very fond of country and western songs and was keen to introduce them. This was not appreciated by the group.

The list of requested songs will, of course, get longer as time goes on. Try to include a combination of regular favourites and new, or less often used, songs.

Be aware of the fact that some songs may trigger particularly painful things for some people. A friend of mine told me that he was once asked not to have 'White

Christmas' in a session as it would have upset a person who had been repeatedly abused as a child to the accompaniment of that very song. In residential settings you may need to be more vigilant about this as the person may not have anyone to explain reasons for their distress. If a song is clearly distressing someone, stop using it.

The nature of the group means that the membership is frequently changing, so you need to be alert to each new member's response to songs.

Finding music

There are many compilations of sheet music. There are music books with songs grouped by era, others by composer and others by type.

Some good examples are:

Essential Songs – The 1930s. Hal Leonard, 2005. ISBN 0881885630

This includes songs such as:

- The Lady Is a Tramp
- My Funny Valentine
- Smoke Gets in Your Eyes
- It's Only a Paper Moon
- On the Sunny Side of the Street
- Red Sails in the Sunset

Essential Songs – The 1940s. Hal Leonard, 2005. ISBN 0634091050

This includes songs such as:

- I Got the Sun in the Morning
- June Is Bustin' Out All Over
- Lili Marlene
- On a Slow Boat to China
- That Old Black Magic

- The White Cliffs of Dover
- Zip-a-Dee-Doo-Dah
- Oh, What a Beautiful Mornin'

Essential Songs – The 1950s. Hal Leonard, 2005. ISBN 0634091042

This includes songs such as:

- Love and Marriage
- Catch a Falling Star
- Magic Moments
- Music! Music! Music!
- Singing the Blues

All of these books include piano music, lyrics and guitar chords.

Another useful source is the Ulverscroft large-print song books. These have many of the tunes you will want to use and the piano parts have been made fairly simple, so if you are not a great pianist you can use this either on the day or, more likely, to play through beforehand to get the melody into your head.

Many music shops have software and copyright allowance to a variety of songs and will print off songs for a small fee. This saves you having to buy a whole book.

Apart from music shops, libraries will be a useful source as well as charity shops.

YouTube and other internet sites can be a great source of materials. Videos on YouTube will often provide examples of style and melody for a song. I have sometimes found this a mixed blessing. Watching Judy Garland sing 'Somewhere Over the Rainbow' or 'The Trolley Song' can only remind me of how brilliant she was and how far short I fall. But I and you need to remember that the purpose of the singing is to enjoy it.

Tempo

You will also need to be aware of whether songs are stimulating or calming.

Try to keep a variety within the session with calmer melodic songs such as 'Somewhere Over the Rainbow' contrasted with something more upbeat such as 'Alexander's Ragtime Band'. It is a good idea to build up to more stimulating songs throughout the session and then towards the end return to calming songs.

Number of songs

The length of the session will determine how many songs you have. The number of songs will also be determined by how often you sing a song through, how many verses you use in some songs, how much talk there is between songs, how able people are to concentrate and how comfortable the chairs are.

It is a good idea to have more songs than you may need. This will allow you to be flexible.

It is also a good idea to divide the session up into three sections. This helps with planning and will mean that the session has some different themes. A quiz can act as a way of dividing up the session.

Musical introductions

Introductions to songs need to be clear so that everyone knows when to start singing. The keyboard player will often lead in by playing the last line of the song. If you have too long an introduction, people will often think they have to start singing and then it is confusing. The leader needs to indicate clearly the moment that the group should join in and start singing.

Introductory stories and anecdotes

It is also a good idea to have some type of verbal introduction to each song. This will help you to pace the sessions and communicate with the group and also gives people a bit of a breather between songs. It should not be more than a few sentences but is often a neat way of focusing on the song. One way to introduce the songs is to give the name of the composer and perhaps a personal link or an anecdote about the song.

This time can be used to speak directly to the participants and can provide a valuable moment to get to know each other, build up relationships, relax all involved and get to know others' tastes in songs and music.

Sometimes I will ask people if they know which musical the song came from and then may say something about the musical.

There are stories about most songs; you just need to find them. A good source is the internet. The information does not have to be lengthy; in fact, too long and people will lose interest.

Short anecdotes, such as the following, work well:

When You're Smiling

Dean Martin, who was known for his enjoyment of a drink, used to say that the song 'When You're Smiling' could just as well be 'When You're Drinking'.

You Made Me Love You

The song was written in 1913 and performed the same year by Al Jolson in *Honeymoon Express*. It was in this song that he first did his characteristic singing position – down on one knee with arms outstretched, a stance later associated with his song 'Mammy'. There is a story that he had an ingrown toenail that was so painful he had to get down on one knee, but to cover up the real reason he stretched out his arms in a dramatic fashion.

Keep Right on to the End of the Road

Harry Lauder wrote 'Keep Right On to the End of the Road' after his only son was killed in the First World War.

Yellow Rose of Texas

This song was published in 1858. It was a song sung during the American Civil War. It was then rarely heard until Mitch Miller made a recording of it in 1950.

Lili Marlene

This song became popular after it was played on Radio Belgrade in 1941. It was heard by troops fighting on both sides of the war in North Africa and Europe. British troops loved it as much as the German troops.

Joseph Goebbels thought the song sentimental and not the sort of thing German troops should be listening to. He tried to ban it. Radio Belgrade received so many letters from soldiers all over Europe asking them to play 'Lili Marlene' that Goebbels reluctantly changed his mind.

The use of percussion instruments

Be very cautious about the use of percussion instruments, especially in care settings where there may not be one carer to each person with dementia and so the instruments get used 'willy-nilly'. This can lead to a cacophony of noise which drowns out the melody.

Percussion instruments should only be handed out if the song really calls for this type of accompaniment and then be taken back, politely, before the next song begins. If they are left with people, some will not realise that they are only to be used with the music and will simply shake, bang, ring them when it is not appropriate, which can be distracting and irritating for others in the group and could lead to some people not attending the group because of the distraction.

It is perhaps best to use instruments with caution or if in doubt leave them out!

Planning a session

The main part of a session may consist of up to 18 songs. This, however, depends on the length of the songs, the setting, the time available and the needs of the participants. The number will also be influenced by how much talk and banter there is between songs and how many rounds, walking and repeat songs are used. It is important here to be flexible. If a song goes well then repeat it. If not, move on and probably do not use it again.

At particular times of the year it is a good idea to have themed songs during the early part of the session. Appendix One will give some example themes.

Be aware that some songs have too many verses. It is generally best to sing a chorus and no more than three verses with plenty of chorus interspersed.

You will see from the sample programmes given later that after about four songs sung in unison it is a good idea to do something different. Then do a few more together and then another change, and so on throughout the session.

When planning a session it can be helpful to think of it in sections. Having three sections seems to work well and below is an example of a session planned in such a way, but there is no reason to see this as a hard and fast rule. For some groups a more organic free-flowing approach may be better. For many groups it will probably be a combination of both approaches, with a structure that can be varied and even abandoned in response to the mood and needs of the group at the time of the session.

Example session structure

Welcoming songs and opening songs

As stated earlier it is a good idea to start off with the same song each time. Any welcoming song will suit. For example:

- Here We Are Again
- Hello, Dolly! (here each person turns to the person next to them and says their name)
- It's a Good Time to Get Acquainted

'It's a Good Time to Get Acquainted' can open the session, but it is a good one to do second. It involves people holding hands with the person or people next to them.

It's a Good Time to Get Acquainted
(Sung to the tune of 'It's a Long Way to Tipperary')
It's a good time to get acquainted,
It's a good time to know
Who is sitting close beside you.
Just smile and say hello.
Goodbye lonesome feeling,
Farewell worldly care,
Here's my hand, my name is ———,
Put YOUR hand right there.

The first section
If appropriate it can be useful to take a theme for this section. Themes might be around festivals, seasons or even something personal that you can link a story to.

- A spring theme might contain:
- I'll Be with You in Apple Blossom Time
- Tulips from Amsterdam
- Tiptoe Through the Tulips
- Easter Bonnet
- I Love Paris in the Springtime

More examples of themed song groups are given in Appendix One.
   The set below I used after I had been on holiday in Torridon, an area of Scotland that is very hilly and has changeable weather. I was walking with a group, hence the 'She'll Be Coming Round the Mountain'. I was able to tell a story that involved all the songs.

- Here We Are Again
- Oh, What a Beautiful Mornin'
- Singing in the Rain
- Somewhere Over the Rainbow
- She'll Be Coming Round the Mountain
- The Happy Wanderer (sing through once, then walk with a partner or partners)

The middle section

I live in Scotland so we always have a number of Scottish songs in this section. You may have particular songs for the place where you live. Scottish songs:

- The Northern Lights of Old Aberdeen
- The River Clyde
- I Belong to Glasgow
- Mairi's Wedding (sing through once, then dance with a partner)
- Loch Lomond

You could also sing songs from a particular musical. For example, *My Fair Lady*:

- I'm Getting Married in the Morning
- Get Me to the Church on Time
- I Could Have Danced All Night
- On the Street Where You Live
- Wouldn't It Be Loverly

It is important, however, not to get hung up on having links and themes. You just need to have good songs that you know everyone likes.

The quiz

Depending on the length of the session it can be both fun and useful to break up the singing a bit. With a small group there is the opportunity to talk to people or tell a story, but with a larger group this can be difficult. One device that offers a break and a change is having a short quiz. This needs to be uncomplicated and should require answers that you are certain people will know.

A useful format for the quiz is for the pianist to play the first few bars of four or five pieces. After the first notes of a song people are invited to call out which song it is. Then move on to the next song. A formula that works is to have songs that have a common theme. For example, all the songs might have:

- A colour in the title
- A season in the title

- Something to do with birds
- A tree in the title
- Something to do with food
- A city in the title
- Something to do with the sky
- 'Night' in the title
- A part of the body in the title

Very often people will then go on to sing the songs unprompted.

The final section

Again a theme is a good idea, but sometimes just having a lot of really good, enjoyable songs that you know people like is what you need here.

Use lyrical, quieter songs towards the end of the session. Songs such as 'Somewhere Over the Rainbow' and 'Edelweiss' are good examples of such songs.

A final section might be as follows:

-
- Waiting at the Church
- Que Sera Sera (divide verses as appropriate between men and women)
- I'm Going to Sit Right Down and Write Myself a Letter
- Something Inside Me Says 'Time for My Tea' (round)
- Edelweiss
- Wish Me Luck as You Wave Me Goodbye

Final song

As with the first song it is a good idea to always have the same song so that people know that this is the end, and the song itself also needs to give that message. Songs such as 'Wish Me Luck as You Wave Me Goodbye' and 'So Long, Farewell' are good ones to use.

As mentioned in Chapter Fourteen, in a residential setting you might not want to emphasise the 'goodbye', so a song such as 'Here's to the Next Time' may be a good idea.

Saying 'goodbye' to everyone
To the tune of 'Goodnight, Ladies' go round the group and shake everyone's hand, singing their name in turn, as follows: 'Goodbye Bill, goodbye Jane, goodbye Arthur, it's time to say goodbye' and so on. Everyone else can join in.

CHAPTER SEVENTEEN

Different formats for variety

You will see that not all songs are sung in unison and that there are some songs with movement involved.

It is a good idea to break up the session with various formats for singing the songs. Different formats will have different purposes and effects. You will need to determine what to use with your group and when by getting to know the members, what they can do and what they enjoy. For rounds and partner songs you will need to have another person helping you. For actions and walking/dancing songs you will need to be aware of the capabilities of participants and also, for the walking songs, have sufficient help from others to support people who may be unsteady on their feet. People in wheelchairs should still be encouraged to join in the movement round the room. Sitting on the sidelines watching others may be a bit lonely.

At the end of this chapter is a summary of the various benefits of using the different song types and formats. This should help with developing a balanced, enjoyable, purposeful and varied session. You can use the following to do this:

- Rounds and canons
- Action songs
- Partner songs
- Call-and-response songs
- Dividing men and women
- Songs to walk or dance to
- A few examples of each of these will be given below.

Rounds and canons

Rounds and canons are well-known formats. Most people will have sung rounds when they were young. They are also a good way to get some lovely harmonies going. Singing a round is a case of follow-my-leader — you sing what you've just heard and, hey presto, there's a counter-melody which is identical to the first melody. The following are a few of the well-known rounds and canons:

• Belle Mama
• Something Inside Me Says 'Time for My Tea'
• Make New Friends
• Frère Jacques
• Three Blind Mice
• London Bridge Is Falling Down
• London's Burning

Beware these last ones as they might sound a bit childish, but I always say how I enjoy them as I can remember doing them at school. I have never come across anyone expressing any discomfort or distaste at singing them.

A round is the same as a canon, except a whole phrase is usually sung before the next voice enters. They're virtually interchangeable, though.

How to do it

First sing the song through in unison. Then divide the group up into two and, if you are brave and the song allows for it, then three. Make this as much fun as possible. I always ask the section I am leading to sing out so that I do not get lulled into singing the other part. Rounds can produce wonderful harmonies and a great sense of achievement when they work. When they don't work they produce a lot of laughter. Do not aim for perfection!

Belle Mama: an example of a round

'Belle Mama' is a beautiful Polynesian song. When sung as a round it results in some lovely harmonies. It also only has two words so it is easy to remember.

Sing through first in unison, maybe two or three times. Then sing in two parts and then, if possible, in four parts. Each new part comes in on the second bar. It is very helpful to have a leader to lead each part. The leaders should also indicate with their hands whether the melody is rising or falling.

BELLE MAMA

TRAD.

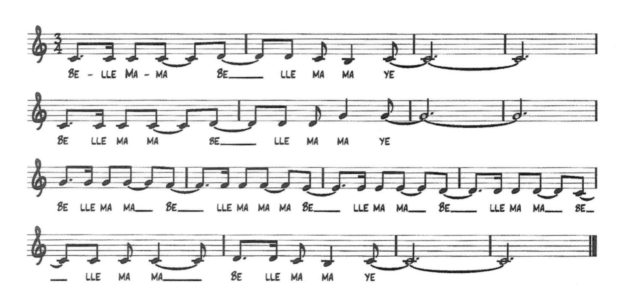

Action songs

These are good ways to get people moving. Increasingly, people with dementia will have problems with purposeful movements such as clapping and touching parts of their body. You will need to judge which actions to use and which might be too demanding.

Music does, of course, move us all. People will sway to music quite naturally and this can be built on. People will also tap their feet and their thighs. Of course clapping can be introduced to most songs and this is a way of getting movement. There is a slight possibility that action songs can become a bit childish; just beware. I find that laughing about them is a good idea. Of course laughter is a good action.

Examples of action songs are:

* My Bonnie Lies Over the Ocean
* On the Sunny Side of the Street
* Do-Re-Mi

My Bonnie Lies Over the Ocean: an example of an action song

Words:
My Bonnie lies over the ocean,
My Bonnie lies over the sea,
My Bonnie lies over the ocean,
O bring back my Bonnie to me.

Chorus:

Bring back, bring back,
Bring back my Bonnie to me, to me,
Bring back, bring back,
O bring back my Bonnie to me.

O blow, ye winds, over the ocean,
And blow the winds over the sea,
O blow the winds over the ocean
And bring back my Bonnie to me.

Chorus

Last night as I lay on my pillow,
Last night as I lay on my bed,
Last night as I lay on my pillow,
I dreamed that my Bonnie was dead.

Chorus

The winds have blown over the ocean,
The winds have blown over the sea,
The winds have blown over the ocean
And brought back my Bonnie to me

Brought back, brought back,
Brought back my Bonnie to me, to me,
Brought back, brought back,
Brought back my Bonnie to me.

Actions to put to the words:

My Bonnie lies over the ocean	For 'My Bonnie' either circle your hand round your face or with both hands outline the shape of a women's body. 'Over the ocean': wave hand and arm in front of you as if they are waves.
My Bonnie lies over the sea	Same as above.
My Bonnie lies over the ocean	Same as above.
O bring back my Bonnie to me	'O bring back': hold arms in front and then bring them back to touch your back. 'To me': point to yourself.
Chorus	All the above as appropriate.
O blow, ye winds, over the ocean	Put hands to mouth as if blowing for 'O blow, ye winds', then do the wave action for the ocean.
Chorus	As previously.
Last night as I lay on my pillow	Hands together to form the pillow and lay head on them to the side.
I dreamed that my Bonnie was dead	Pull a long face.
Chorus	
Last verse and Chorus	As above.

Partner songs

These always give a great sense of achievement when they work and lots of laughter when they don't. First sing each song through at least once and then allocate a song to each side of the circle. It is a good idea to have two leaders/conductors for this. People can then be told which person they are to look at and follow.

Once you have sung them through, sing them in tandem. Once that has worked you can sing them through twice.

Songs that work include:

- 'It's a Long Way to Tipperary' and 'Pack Up Your Troubles' (you need to make sure that the group singing 'It's a Long Way to Tipperary' sing 'It's' before the other group come in!)
- 'Michael Finnegan' and 'Bobby Shafto'
- 'What Shall We Do with the Drunken Sailor?' and 'Sinner Man'
- 'Swing Low, Sweet Chariot' and 'When the Saints Go Marching In' (for this one the group singing 'When the Saints' have to start and when they sing 'saints', the group singing 'Swing Low, Sweet Chariot' come in, so 'saints' and 'swing' will be sung together)

Bobby Shafto and Michael Finnegan

Bobby Shafto has gone to sea, Silver buckles on his knee. He'll come back and marry me, Bonny Bobby Shafto.	There once was a man named Michael Finnegan. He grew whiskers on his chinnigin. The wind came down and blew them in again. Poor old Michael Finnegan.

Call-and-response songs

Divide the group into two. It is a good idea to have two people leading this. Participants can then be told which person to follow. If doing this on your own then you need to be emphatic about who sings when, turning your body towards the group you want to sing.

Some examples of call-and-response songs:

- The Banana Boat Song
- There Is a Tavern in the Town
- Polly Wolly Doodle
- Oh Dear, What Can the Matter Be?
- Oh Happy Day
- Gilly Gilly Ossenfeffer Katzenellenbogen by the Sea.
- Down by the Riverside

'Down by the Riverside' has many verses and it would be too much to do all of them. You will need to decide how many to do, depending on your group. It is good to get someone to shout out 'where' each time before the responding group sing 'Down by the riverside'.

Dividing men and women

So long as there are enough men this can be amusing.
- Que Sera Sera (the men sing the verse 'when I was just a little boy' and the women 'when I was just a little girl', everyone sings the other verses)
- I'd Do Anything
- Daisy Daisy (the men sing 'Daisy Daisy' and the women sing the second verse 'Henry Henry')

Daisy Daisy: an example of dividing men and women

Sing through once, then divide into men and women.

> **Men:** Daisy, Daisy, give me your answer do.
> I'm half-crazy all for the love of you.
> It won't be a stylish marriage,
> I can't afford a carriage.
> But you'll look sweet
> Upon the seat
> Of a bicycle made for two.

> **Women:** Henry, Henry, this is my answer true.
> I'm not crazy, oh, for the love of you.
> If you can't afford a carriage,
> Forget about the marriage.
> I won't be jammed,
> I won't be crammed
> On a bicycle made for two.

Walking/dancing songs

These are always very popular. Walking songs can be used for walking, swaying, rocking, clapping, shoulder movements, swinging arms.

There is, of course, a need to be careful about supporting people who are experiencing difficulties with mobility and balance. It is often important to have one person on each side of the person with dementia. Also people using wheelchairs can be pushed round or some will just stand up and sway. It is important to emphasise that some people might want to 'sit this out' but they can still sing along. It is a good idea to have someone with people who sit it out and maybe they can hold hands and sway.

Examples of songs to walk to:

- Mairi's Wedding
- The Happy Wanderer
- Side by Side
- Keep Right On to the End of the Road
- Strolling (Flanagan and Allen)
- Tiptoe Through the Tulips
- On the Sunny Side of the Street
- Lambeth Walk

A sample list of songs to dance to can be found in Appendix One.

Summary of the different formats and their benefits

SONG FORMAT/TYPE	INVOLVES	BENEFIT
Opening songs	Same song/s each session	Familiarises participants with the format/expectations of the session. Promotes group feeling. May encourage identity of group, perhaps by using local song, e.g. 'I'm a Lassie from Lancashire'.
Themed songs	For example: songs from a show, Christmas songs	Aids recognition and continuity. Enables a story to be woven through the songs, related to e.g. a musical or a season or holiday.

SONG FORMAT/TYPE	INVOLVES	BENEFIT
Rounds	Singing a song in parts, from simple to quite complex	Creates sense of achievement when it works. Encourages laughter when it doesn't work. Can create some lovely harmonies. These should be commented on. Enables greater involvement of carers.
Partner songs	A different song for each side of the circle sung at the same time	Promotes achievement, competition and laughter.
Call-and-response	Songs requiring question and answer	For some participants this is easier than straight lyrics as they are prompted for the answer. Enables some to participate when difficult at other times. People may look at other people in the group rather than the leader. This helps with group feelings of belonging and involvement.
Dividing men and women		Encourages fun of competition. Can enable more direct contact e.g. between a male participant and female carer or vice versa

SONG FORMAT/TYPE	INVOLVES	BENEFIT
Walking/dancing songs	For those able, walking and dancing or more hand/body movements	Movement stimulates the body, brain and emotions. Promotes interest and motivation. Involves contact with others. Often after the walking/ dancing songs the group will sing even more lustily.
Final section	Rousing songs	Creates enjoyment and sense of achievement. Aids breathing and muscle use.
Finale songs	Quieter songs Same finishing song each session	Helps people to wind down. Promotes understanding that the session is ending.

CHAPTER EIGHTEEN

Sample programmes

These are offered as a way to get started. Every group will develop its own favourites and style. I am not suggesting that these are the best but offer them as examples of what has worked.

Examples are given of programmes from community groups, an early onset group and residential/nursing home groups.

Community group programmes

Programme 1

Welcome and warm-up

First section

- Here We Are Again
- Getting to Know You
- I'm Getting Married in the Morning
- Waiting at the Church
- I'm Going to Sit Right Down and Write Myself a Letter
- Side by Side (once though and then walk)
- When You're Smiling
- Belle Mama (once through, then as a round)

Middle section: songs associated with Judy Garland

- Meet Me in St Louis
- Somewhere Over the Rainbow
- The Trolley Song
- The Wizard of Oz

Quiz

Four songs associated with the colour red (play the first few notes and people guess the song):

- Red Sails in the Sunset
- When the Red, Red Robin
- A Red, Red Rose
- Rudolph the Red-Nosed Reindeer

Final section

- Alexander's Ragtime Band
- Swing Low, Sweet Chariot
- When the Saints Go Marching In

Sing previous two songs as partner songs

- Edelweiss
- Wish Me Luck as You Wave Me Goodbye

Goodbye to everyone

Programme 2: songs for spring

Welcome and warm-up

First section

- Here We Are Again
- I Love Paris in the Springtime
- Tulips from Amsterdam
- Oh, What a Beautiful Mornin'
- Tiptoe Through the Tulips (sing through, then walk/dance)
- Easter Bonnet

Middle section: Scottish songs

- The Northern Lights of Old Aberdeen
- A Gordon for Me
- I Belong to Glasgow
- Mairi's wedding (sing through once, then walk)
- Loch Lomond

Quiz

Four songs associated with rivers (play the first few notes and people guess the song):

- Sailing Down the River
- Moon River
- The Song of the Clyde
- Old Man River

Final section

- Down by the Riverside (call and response)
- Don't Sit Under the Apple Tree
- Keep Right On to the End of the Road (sometimes this can be good to stand and march on the spot to)
- Alexander's Ragtime Band
- Somewhere Over the Rainbow
- We'll Gather Lilacs
- Wish Me Luck as You Wave Me Goodbye

Goodbye song

Programme 3

Welcome and warm-up

- Hello, Dolly! (saying the name of the person next to you)
- Little Brown Jug
- When the Red, Red Robin
- Red Roses for a Blue Lady
- Scarlet Ribbons
- Make New Friends (round)
- Yellow Rose of Texas
- Tie a Yellow Ribbon
- You Are My Sunshine
- All Things Bright and Beautiful
- Smilin' Through
- Step We Gaily (promenade)
- I Love a Lassie
- The Wild Mountain Thyme
- Michael Finnegan/This Old Man (partner songs)

- Edelweiss
- What a Wonderful World
- Somewhere Over the Rainbow
- As We Go Now

Programme 4

Welcome and warm-up

First section

- Here We Are Again
- It's a Good Time to Get Acquainted
- Nice Cup of Tea
- My Favourite Things
- Make New Friends (round)
- Happy Talk
- The Bells Are Ringing (sing through, then walk)

Middle section

- Alexander's Ragtime Band
- On the Sunny Side of the Street
- What Shall We Do with the Drunken Sailor?/Sinner Man (partner songs)
- In Dublin's Fair City
- The Wild Rover

Quiz

Four songs associated with parts of the body (play the first few notes and people guess the song):

- You Need Hands
- Jeannie with the Light Brown Hair
- The Hokey Cokey (you put your right leg in etc.)
- Knees Up Mother Brown

Final section

- Mother Kelly's Doorstep
- You Made Me Love You
- Side by Side (sing through, then walk)
- Belle Mama (sing through twice, not as a round)
- We'll Meet Again
- Wish Me Luck as You Wave Me Goodbye

Goodbye song

Programme for a small early onset group

Welcome and warm-up

- I Believe for Every Drop of Rain That Falls
- Streets of London
- Don't Dilly Dally (My Old Man)
- If You Were the Only Girl in the World
- The Wonder of You
- The Wild Rover
- Daisy Daisy/Henry Henry (divide men and women)

- You'll Never Walk Alone
- Loch Lomond
- Consider Yourself
- Imagine
- I'll Be Your Sweetheart
- Beautiful Dreamer
- Swing Low, Sweet Chariot/When the Saints Go Marching In (sung separately, then as partner songs)
- Somewhere Over the Rainbow
- Bye Bye Blackbird

Programmes for homes for older people

You will see that these programmes do not include any walking about; this is because the room in the home is not sufficiently large. Generally the people in these groups are more frail than the people in the community and so would need more support even if walking were possible. These programmes are all with songs sung in unison.

Programme 1

Programme for St Patrick's Day

Welcome and warm-up

First section

- Here We Are Again
- Hello, Hello, Who's Your Lady Friend?
- When You're Smiling
- The Happy Wanderer

Middle section: Irish songs

- When Irish Eyes Are Smiling
- If You're Irish
- It's a Long Way to Tipperary
- McNamara's Band
- The Wild Rover (remember the clapping)
- Danny Boy
- Cockles and Mussels
- I'll Take You Home Again, Kathleen
- Galway Bay

Quiz

What is the colour we associate with Ireland? *Green.*

Songs with 'green' in the title (play the first few notes and people guess the song):

- Green Door
- Greensleeves
- Green Green Grass of Home
- Ten Green Bottles
- Green Grow the Rushes, O!

Final section

- Roamin' in the Gloamin'
- Charlie Is My Darling
- I Love a Lassie
- Wish Me Luck as You Wave Me Goodbye
- Goodbye, Ladies

Programme 2

Welcome and warm-up

- Here We Are Again

First section: London songs

- Lambeth Walk
- My Old Man
- I'm Henery the Eighth, I Am
- Maybe It's Because I'm a Londoner
- I'm Getting Married in the Morning

Middle section: sunshine songs

- You Are My Sunshine
- The Sun Has Got His Hat On
- When You're Smiling
- Happy Days Are Here Again

Quiz

Songs associated with birds (play the first few notes and people guess the song):

- Bye Bye Blackbird
- Chick Chick Chicken
- A Nightingale Sang in Berkeley Square
- There'll Be Bluebirds Over the White Cliffs of Dover

Final section: Scottish songs, animal songs, farewell songs

- Donald, Where's Your Troosers?
- I Belong to Glasgow
- Mairi's Wedding
- Skye Boat Song
- Daddy Wouldn't Buy Me a Bow-Wow
- How Much Is That Doggy in the Window?
- We'll Meet Again
- Good-bye-ee!
- Goodnight, Ladies

Programme 3

Welcome and warm-up

- Here We Are Again

First section: flower songs

- Tiptoe Through the Tulips
- Tulips from Amsterdam
- Roses of Picardy
- Scarborough Fair
- We'll Gather Lilacs

Second section: songs with names in the title

- K-K-K-Katy
- Joshua
- Jeannie with the Light Brown Hair
- I'm Just Wild About Harry
- Goodbye, Dolly Gray
- Lili Marlene

Quiz

Songs about rain and weather (play the first few notes and people guess the song):

- Singin' in the Rain
- Stormy Weather
- Raindrops Keep Fallin' on My Head
- Somewhere Over the Rainbow
- Blow the Wind Southerly
- You'll Never Walk Alone

Final section: love and marriage songs, farewell songs

- Daisy Daisy followed by Henry Henry
- Get Me to the Church on Time
- I'm Henery the Eighth, I Am
- Ma, He's Making Eyes at Me
- The Bells Are Ringing
- Goodnight, Sweetheart
- Good-bye-ee!
- Goodnight, Ladies

Appendices

Themes for song combinations

Flowers

Tiptoe Through the Tulips
Tulips from Amsterdam
I'll Be with You in Apple Blossom Time
We'll Gather Lilacs
Roses of Picardy
A Red, Red Rose
You Are My Honeysuckle

Travels

Wonderful Copenhagen
The Happy Wanderer
I Love Paris
The Streets of London
I Belong to Glasgow
Oklahoma
Arrivederci Roma
In Dublin's Fair City
Tulips from Amsterdam
Eviva España

Seasons

Autumn Leaves
Winter Wonderland
It Might as Well Be Spring
June is Bustin' Out All Over
When It's Spring Again
Easter Bonnet
Summer Holiday

Boys' names

Charlie Is My Darling
Oh Johnny, Oh Johnny, Oh!
John Peel
Billy Boy
Michael Finnegan
Oliver
Walter, Walter, Lead Me to the Altar

Girls' names

Sally
Daisy Daisy
K-K-K-Katy
Dinah
Charmaine
Barbara Allen
Eleanor Rigby
Delilah

Songs from musicals

The King and I

Getting to Know You
Hello, Young Lovers
I Whistle a Happy Tune
Shall We Dance?
Something Wonderful
We Kiss in a Shadow

State Fair

It Might as Well Be Spring
It's a Grand Night for Singing

South Pacific

Bali Ha'i
Dites-Moi
Happy Talk
There is Nothing Like a Dame
This Nearly Was Mine
Wonderful Guy
Some Enchanted Evening
Younger than Springtime
I'm Gonna Wash That Man Right Out of My Hair

My Fair Lady

Get Me to the Church on Time
I Could Have Danced All Night
I've Grown Accustomed to Your Face
On the Street Where You Live
The Rain in Spain
With a Little Bit of Luck
Wouldn't It Be Loverly

The Sound of Music

Sixteen Going on Seventeen
Do-Re-Mi
Climb Every Mountain
Edelweiss
My Favourite Things
The Sound of Music

Oklahoma
People Will Say We're in Love
The Surrey with the Fringe on Top
Out of My Dreams
Oh, What a Beautiful Mornin'
I Cain't Say No

Carousel

If I Loved You
June Is Bustin' Out All Over
You'll Never Walk Alone

Songs to dance to or use different tempos with

The songs below are ones used in a sheltered housing complex where the people are generally more mobile and many still want to dance to the songs. A couple of these are built into each programme.

Anniversary Song (waltz)
Are You Lonesome Tonight? (waltz)
Bill Bailey (quickstep)
Chanson D'Amour (shuffle)
Hokey Cokey (party time)
Danny Boy (foxtrot)
Deep in the Heart of Texas (2/4 march)
Happy Days Are Here Again (quickstep)
Have You Ever Been Lonely? (foxtrot)
Lambeth Walk (party time)
McNamara's Band (6/8 march)
Memories Are Made of This (quickstep)
Slow Boat to China (foxtrot)
Rock Around the Clock (rock)
Too Young (foxtrot)
Underneath the Arches (foxtrot)
We'll Meet Again (foxtrot)
You Are My Sunshine (quickstep)
You're Nobody Till Somebody Loves You (foxtrot)

A sample constitution

THE SINGING GROUP AT ....

AIMS

1. To seek to improve the quality of life for people with dementia and their carers through social and musical engagement.
2. To help heighten self-esteem and relieve isolation.

OBJECTIVES

1. To provide an enjoyable experience for people with dementia and their carers.
2. To provide an opportunity for people with dementia to engage in an activity that is known to provide suitable stimulation.
3. To enable people with dementia to engage in an activity that focuses on their retained skills.
4. To provide an activity that will help to reduce agitation and distress.
5. To provide a forum where people with dementia and their carers can socialise with others who share their concerns and challenges.
6. To provide appropriate information and support.
7. To ensure that confidentiality is held in all matters relating to the group's members and carers. Any queries or concerns should be referred to the Management Committee.

ACTIVITIES

1. The group will be run [frequency].
2. The group will be staffed by volunteers, all of whom will have training on

dementia and will demonstrate an understanding of the needs of people with dementia and their carers.

3. Volunteers and in particular the Management Committee will organise fundraising events.

POWERS

1. The Management Committee will have the power to do anything which is calculated to further its aims, objectives and activities.

MEMBERSHIP

Membership includes people with dementia and their carers, and volunteers who support the running of the sessions.

Criteria for membership

Membership is open to:

- Anyone with dementia accompanied by their carer/s.
- Volunteers who demonstrate an empathy with and understanding of the needs of people with dementia and their carers.

Membership – rules and restrictions:

- Membership is free.
- The decision to accept people into the group is the responsibility of the Management Committee.
- There are no restrictions on membership for people with dementia and their carers unless there is an issue of health and safety, in relation to their needs.
- Potential members or their carer/s will approach a member of the Management Committee to discuss joining the group.
- Potential volunteer members will approach a member of the Management Committee to discuss their contribution and attendance.

- Volunteers must be willing to undertake an afternoon's training on dementia. This is provided by members of the Management Committee.
- Volunteers would be refused membership if it was decided that they did not have the understanding needed to support people with dementia and their carers. Membership would be ended if they breached confidentiality or engaged in other behaviours considered inappropriate or detrimental to the support and wellbeing of people with dementia and their carers.

GENERAL MEETING OF MEMBERS

- An annual general meeting (AGM) will be held each year close to the anniversary of the beginning of the group.
- All members will be informed by e-mail and by word of mouth.

The AGM will address pertinent issues including:

1. The financial position.
2. How moneys have been raised and spent over the previous year.
3. The learning from the past year in relation to the way the singing group has developed.
4. Ideas for improving the experience of the group.
5. Identifying any problems, and trying to find solutions.
6. Any other current business.

- If there is need for additional general meetings, all members will be notified of these by both e-mail and word of mouth.
- There will need to be six members of the group at an AGM for it to be quorate.
- The meeting will be run by a member of the Management Committee.
- Decisions will be taken by discussions leading to consensus. Where this is not achieved a vote will be taken of all members who attend the meeting. The Management Committee will be bound by such decisions taken at AGM.

MANAGEMENT OF THE GROUP

* The group will have a management committee.
* This will be called 'The Singing Group Management Committee', hereafter called the Committee.
* The Committee will have four to six members.
* Any group member with appropriate skills and experience can be on the Committee.
* Committee members will be chosen depending on the needs of the group and the skills of the individual.
* Anyone with relevant information and expertise on any area required to run the group will be permitted to attend Committee meetings.
* Membership of the Committee will be reviewed after five years.
* If a member leaves prior to five years' service another member of the group will be asked to join.
* The Committee will meet as and when necessary but not less than six times a year.
* Meetings will be conducted by rotation amongst the Committee members.
* The minimum number of Committee members needed for the meeting to be valid is three.
* Two members will be designated as treasurers and will be responsible for financial affairs. These people will volunteer for this role.
* The Management Committee will keep other members of the group informed of their decisions by word of mouth, e-mail and written account to be presented at AGM.

The Committee is responsible for:

* the running of the singing sessions
* issuing and maintaining volunteer agreements
* maintaining the standard of quality of the delivery of the sessions
* determining criteria for volunteers
* accepting or rejecting volunteers
* maintaining the standard required of volunteers

- the provision of training to volunteers
- coordinating the various activities such as provision of refreshments, fundraising, special events etc.
- the management of administration and finances
- carrying out the wishes of the membership expressed through decisions taken at AGM
- publicity, development and outreach

MONEY AND PROPERTY

- Money is kept in a bank account. Two named members of the Committee have authority to sign any transactions with the full agreement of the Committee.
- Information about accounts will be made available at Committee meetings and to all members at the AGM.
- A suitably qualified independent person will be appointed to check and independently scrutinise the accounts.
- Payment of expenses and other payments will be ratified by the Committee.
- Property held on behalf of the Committee will be held in rotation by members of the Committee.

CHANGING THE CONSTITUTION

- Rules of the constitution can only be changed after discussion within the Committee and ratified at the AGM, by at least two thirds of the members present and eligible to vote.
- All changes have to be ratified at the AGM.
- Two aspects of the constitution which cannot be changed are: the criteria for becoming accepted as a volunteer, and decisions made by the Committee regarding membership.

CLOSING THE GROUP DOWN

- Any decision to close the group down would be made following discussion within the Committee and at the AGM. At least two thirds of the members present and eligible to vote at the AGM must agree.
- Disposal of the group's assets which remain after closing down would be by gifting them to another organisation with similar aims and objectives. The final AGM of the group would determine which similar organisation will benefit.

[date]

An outline plan for preparing and running a session

You may want to base the structure of your first sessions on the following outline. Insert your choice of songs and quiz using the sample programmes provided. You will soon develop the most appropriate programmes for your group.

Example of a session plan

TASK	WHO	WHEN	COMMENTS/WHY/ISSUES
PREPARATIONS 1. Check venue	Jo Bloggs	Each week/3 days before session?	See Part Two, 'Preparing to Get Started'.
2. Check volunteers	Bill Bailey	Each week/3 days before session?	Who? How many? Allocate roles. See Part Two.
3. Notify/remind participants/institution of next session date	Sally Smith	Previous session/3 days before?	See Part Two.
4. Check refreshments	Jill Jones	Come prepared	See Part Two.

TASK	WHO	WHEN	COMMENTS/WHY/ ISSUES
WELCOME 1. Access/entry	Jo Bloggs	Half-hour before	Ensure venue opened and access OK. Ensure accommodation free of other residents/users if group is in residential or day care setting.
2. Refreshments	Jill Jones	On entry	
3. Introductions and welcome	Session leader	When all in position	See Part Two.
WARM-UPS 1. Physical	Session leader? Jo Bloggs?	Start	See Chapter Fifteen, 'Choosing warm-up exercises'.
2. Breathing /voice	Session leader	Total 5 mins	
SECTION ONE Opening songs	Session leader	Dependent on how many and what but estimate time, e.g 10 mins	See Chapter Sixteen, 'Choosing Songs', and the sample programmes in Chapter Eighteen.

TASK	WHO	WHEN	COMMENTS/WHY/ ISSUES
MIDDLE SECTION Themed or favourite songs. Possibly rounds or partner songs etc.	Session leader	As above, estimate time, e.g. 15 mins. May vary based on involvement, enjoyment.	See Chapters Sixteen to Eighteen.
THE QUIZ/GAME	Sally Smith	If time? If enjoyed by participants? Example time: 5 mins	See Chapters Sixteen and Eighteen.
FINAL SECTION Enjoyable ending songs concluding in slower wind-down	Session leader	Need to keep to strict ending time for transport etc. and also concentration ability of participants. Example time: 10 mins	See Chapters Sixteen to Eighteen.
GOODBYE 1. Goodbye to everyone 2. Help participants leave 3. Clear venue	Session leader and support Volunteers/staff Volunteers/staff Jo Bloggs?		See Chapter Sixteen.

References

Aldridge, D (2000). *Music Therapy in Dementia Care*. London: Jessica Kingsley Publishers

Beck, R J, T C Cesario, A Yousefi and H Enamoto (2000). 'Choral Singing, Performance Perception and Immune System Changes in Salivary Immunoglobulin A and Cortisol'. *Musical Perception* 18(1), pp.87–106

Buijssen, H (2005). *The Simplicity of Dementia*. London: Jessica Kingsley Publishers

Casby, J A, and M B Holm (1994). 'The effect of music on repetitive disruptive vocalisations of persons with dementia'. *American Journal of Occupational Therapy* 48(10), pp.883–889

Clair, A A (1991). 'Music therapy for severely regressed persons with probable diagnosis of Alzheimer's disease'. In K Bruscia (ed.), *Case Studies in Music Therapy*. Pheonixville, PA: Barcelona Publishers, pp.571–580

Clair, A A (1996). *Therapeutic Uses of Music with Older Adults*. Baltimore, MD: Health Professions Press

Denney, A (1997). 'Quiet music. An intervention for mealtime agitation?' *Journal of Gerontological Nursing* 23(7), pp.16–23

Levitin, D (2006). *This is Your Brain on Music*. London: Atlantic Books

Nietzsche, F (1888/1974). *The Gay Science*. Translated by Walter Kaufmann. New York: Vintage Books

Noice, T, H Noice and A F Kramer (2013). 'Participatory Arts for Older People: A Review of Benefits and Challenges'. *The Gerontologist*

Ortiz, J M (1997). *The Tao of Music*. Newburyport, MA: Weiser Books

Ragneskog, H, G Brane, I Karlsson and M Kihlgren (1996). 'Influence of dinner music on food intake and symptoms common to dementia'. *Scandinavian Journal of Caring Science* 10(1), pp.11–17

Rio, R (2009). *Connecting through Music with People with Dementia*. London: Jessica Kingsley Publishers

Sacks, O (2007). *Musicophilia*. London: Picador

Schopenhauer, A (1819/1969). *The World as Will and Representation*. Translated by E F J Payne. New York: Dover

Valentine, E, and C Evans (2001). 'The effects of solo singing, choral singing and swimming on mood and physiological indices'. *British Journal of Medical Psychology* 74, pp.115–120

Vickhoff, B (2013). 'Music structure determines heart rate variability of singers'. *Frontiers in Psychology* 4, p.334

Welch, G (2010). 'The Impact of Singing: An Independent Research-based Evaluation – The story so far'. International Music Research Centre, Institute of Education, University of London

Useful organisations, information and literature

Alzheimer's Society (UK):
Devon House
58 St Katharine's Way
London
E1W 1LB
www.alzheimers.org.uk

Alzheimer Scotland
22 Drumsheugh Gardens
Edinburgh
EH3 7RN
Tel: 0131 243 1453
www.alzscot.org
Email: info@alzscot.org

The Alzheimer Society of Ireland
National Office
Temple Road
Blackrock
Co. Dublin
Tel: (01) 207 3800
www.alzheimer.ie

Dementia Services Development Centre
Iris Murdoch Building
University of Stirling
FK9 4LA
Tel: 01786 467740
www.dementia.stir.ac.uk

Alzheimer's Australia: www.fightdementia.org.au
Alzheimer Society Canada: www.alzheimer.ca
Alzheimer's Association (USA): www.alz.org
Nordoff Robbins Music Therapy Charity: www.nordoff-robbins.org.uk
Performing Rights Society for Music (PRS): www.prsformusic.com

Publications

Journal of Dementia Care. http://www.careinfo.org/journal-of-dementia-care/
The dementia guide (2013). Publ. Alzheimer's Society UK
Caring for the person with dementia: A handbook for families and other carers (2011). Publ. Alzheimer's Society UK
It's me Grandma! It's me! (2010) Storybook for 7–11-year-olds about how a family can be affected by dementia. Publ. Alzheimer's Society Uk
Each day is different: An introduction to the care and support of people with dementia (2009). A beginner's guide to working with people with dementia which provides practical tips and helpful advice for professionals starting out in dementia care. Publ. Alzheimer's Society UK
Activities to Do with Your Parent Who Has Alzheimer's Dementia (2014). Judith Levy. Publ. Amazon CreateSpace
Connecting through Music with People with Dementia: A Guide for Caregivers (2009). Robin Rio. Publ. Jessica Kingsley Publishers
Darkness in the Afternoon (2006). DVD. Publ. Dementia Services Development Centre, University of Stirling

About the author

Diana has a lifelong interest and involvement in music making and has been advocating the use of music with people with dementia for many years. She is now involved with the provision of singing groups for people with dementia.

Diana has over 30 years' experience as a practitioner, researcher, educator and trainer in the field of dementia and learning disability and dementia.

Previously Diana was the Course Director for the MSc in Dementia Studies at the University of Stirling. She was then Research Fellow at the Centre for Research on Families and Relationships at the University of Edinburgh where her area of research and emphasis was predominantly in the field of dementia and learning disability and dementia.

She was also an Associate Consultant to Hammond Care Australia where she provided consultation in learning disability and dementia and on night-time care for people with dementia.

Diana is an advisor to service providers and planners who support people with dementia and people with a learning disability and dementia.

Diana is widely published on topics related to dementia, learning disability and dementia, and night-time care. Her work has been translated into a number of languages including Chinese, Polish, Dutch and Spanish.

She lives in Edinburgh.

CPSIA information can be obtained at www.ICGtesting.com
Printed in the USA
LVOW09s1720290715

448106LV00010B/435/P